A GUT REACTION

A GUT REACTION

*A True Story About a
Mother's Fight to Save her Son's
Life and his Amazing Recovery
from Crohn's Disease*

Sky Curtis

INANNA PUBLICATIONS AND EDUCATION INC.
TORONTO, CANADA

Canada Council for the Arts   **Conseil des Arts du Canada**   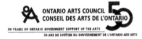

We gratefully acknowledge the support of the Canada Council for the Arts and the Ontario Arts Council for our publishing program. We also acknowledge the financial support of the Ontario Media Development Organization.

We are also grateful for the support received from an Anonymous Fund at The Calgary Foundation.

Library and Archives Canada Cataloguing in Publication

Curtis, Sky, author
    A gut reaction : a true story about a mother's fight to save her son's life and his amazing recovery from Crohn's disease / Sky Curtis.

Issued in print and electronic formats.
ISBN 978-1-77133-080-0 (pbk.). — ISBN 978-1-77133-081-7 (pdf)

    1. Curtis, Sky. 2. Curtis, Sky—Family. 3. Crohn's disease—Patients—Canada—Biography. 4. Crohn's disease—Popular works. I. Title.

RC862.E52C87 2013   362.196'3440092   C2013-902595-2
     C2013-902596-0

Printed and bound in Canada

    MIX
Paper from
responsible sources
FSC® C004071

Inanna Publications and Education Inc.
210 Founders College, York University
4700 Keele Street, Toronto, Ontario, Canada M3J 1P3
Telephone: (416) 736-5356 Fax: (416) 736-5765
Email: inanna.publications@inanna.ca Website: www.inanna.ca

*This book is dedicated with love
to my children*

CONTENTS

FOREWORD

ANY PATIENT WITH chronic ulcerative colitis or Crohn's colitis will be able to explain to the lay person who does have the disease that they are suffering on a daily basis with chronic abdominal pain, cramping, urgency to run to the bathroom, frequent bleeding, weight loss, tiredness, multiple drug therapies with their own side effects, hospitalizations, colonoscopies, biopsies, pathology and drug costs, which become the ever-consuming life of the patient. It can take over the patient's life leaving him/her little time for work, hobbies or pleasure. It is in this context that Chris Curtis, supported valiantly by his mother Sky, took on the battle against a condition that has no known specific cause. Not only did they take on the battle against the disease itself but also against the 'Establishment,' which has in its mind the understanding that colitis is somehow caused by an abnormal reaction to the flora that is normally housed in the bowel. In fact, the whole story revolves around bowel contents. This book is about bowel contents itself. How it protects us. How it can be infected. How the infection can affect the life of the person who is carrying the infected bowel flora. And how this can be corrected.

The human bowel flora contains a complex population of bacteria of several hundred different species. This is a minimum estimate. As each day passes more bacteria are identified by the new genetic methods. The colon itself is densely populated with at least 500 species and more than 30,000 sub-species with their various normal bacteria. Indeed our "poo is a zoo" as it contains many little living animals that live within our bowel. These organisms and the chemicals they produce, can affect the body in a positive or negative sense. This is called the human microbiota. It protects us from invasion by bad bacteria by having a characteristic termed in the late 1980s as being "colonization resistance." If we did not have this resistance then the food we ingest every day, which is relatively polluted by various bacteria as well as viruses, and at times can pass through the gastric acid and the duodenal pancreatic juices—would certainly infect us on a daily basis, giving us chronic diarrhea, pain, gas, cramping and perhaps weight loss. However, we are endowed with a normal bowel flora with enormous numbers of bacteria that prevent implantation. Hence the good bacteria prevent the bowel flora from catching chronic infection. If one considers the bowel flora as a large organ of the body, it too can suffer from various disorders such as infection. Common infections we know are Salmonella, Shigella, Campylobacter and, of course, the epidemic of Clostridium difficile which is well known in North America.

What is less known is that colitis comprises a number of different types of infections that we have not yet identified. Just as one can use normal human flora implanted into the colon to clear up infection of Clostridium difficile, Sky Curtis felt that such implantation of normal flora into Chris's bowel may help clear up his colitis infection.

The use of healthy human flora to implant into the colon would clearly be the most complete probiotic therapy available today. There is no known probiotic available today to mankind that comes close to matching the complexity of the normal human flora. It acts as a broad-spectrum antibiotic factory capable of eradicating bad bacteria and spores because in itself it produces bacteriocins or antibiotic-like agents. Indeed, few people realize that bacteria themselves are the source of many of our normal antibiotics such as Vancomycin, which originated from a bacterium found in Borneo in '50s. Faecal bacteriotherapy or more recently Faecal Microbiota Transplantation (FMT) involves the infusion of healthy human donor faecal slurry or bacteria into the bowel of the recipient who might have the infection causing his illness. It can be dramatically curative in conditions such as recurrent Clostridium difficile infection. However, little work has been done in the area of Ulcerative colitis and Crohn's disease. It can be affective in Irritable Bowel Syndrome—both diarrhea-predominant and constipation-predominant—and there have been some reports of patients who had short-term benefit when colitis was treated.

Sky and Chris Curtis took the disease on. They had the courage and conviction that if a normal bowel flora environment was created recurrently in Chris's bowel then perhaps his colon—which was sentenced to be removed—might reverse its inflammation by killing off the infection with the normal incoming bacteria. Through perseverance, and many minor complications but with the vision of a normal bowel function, Sky and Chris won. This book, *A Gut Reaction*, describes the experience of Sky Curtis and her son Chris using faecal transplantations, under my very distant guidance from Australia, to heal the symptoms and signs of severe colitis as evidenced by absence of active inflammation on a follow-up colonoscopy.

Dr. Thomas J. Borody
Director, Centre for Digestive Diseases
Sydney, Australia

1.

THE BEGINNING

MY SUNBURNED FOURTEEN-YEAR-OLD son was shuffling through the sliding doors at Toronto International Airport, satchel flung over his shoulder. When did he become so tall? So gangly? He was glowering. I could hear his inner thoughts.

I hate my life.

Typical. Oh the joys of being fourteen. He'd just arrived from a holiday in Greece with his grandparents and was now pressing impatiently against the much too slow crowd toward the exit. I leaned over the railing and waved at him excitedly, hoping to catch his eye. As he came closer and into focus I could see that Chris looked different. Very different.

My youngest child was covered in acne. What? I looked again. How did that happen? I had sent him away just two weeks ago with cheeks as smooth as silk, and here he was, covered in zits? What had he eaten? I plastered a smile on my face and tried to look normal.

I gave him a great big hug and mustered up a chuckle. "I'm so glad you're home. Did you have fun?"

He looked at me with the tightened lips of a kid who hadn't been fooled.

"I *know*," he muttered as he turned his face away.

I said to the back of his head, "We'll get you to a doctor, right away. There's good medication for that."

Three years and many bottles of pills and lotions later, Chris was still covered in acne. It hadn't really held him back. He was the first French horn in the orchestra at his high school He was the lead in the play productions. He had a wicked sense of humour and got along with everyone. His friends on Facebook numbered in the thousands. He was Vice-President of the Student Council and raised tons of money for the school by promoting events. He even passed math. He led children on canoe trips into the wilderness. He was affectionate and kind. Chris was not held back by his complexion.

But still. He had acne. The dermatologist, at the end of his rope, finally recommended Accutane, the strongest medication there was on the market for this particular skin condition.

Chris, now at the age of seventeen, sat stoically in front of the doctor as he was warned of all the side effects of this wonder drug. He held the blister pack of pills in his hand and fumbled with the fancy packaging as the doctor's voice droned on and on. I could tell he was only listening with half an ear because he barely snickered as he promised to not get pregnant. He put on his reliable face as he said he would not miss appointments. He earnestly affirmed that if he felt suicidal he'd talk to someone.

I sat with my hands in my lap and listened to the exchange with growing alarm. What kind of drug was this?

I ventured, "This drug sounds pretty scary. Is it safe?"

The dermatologist turned toward me dismissively. "It's a

derivative from Vitamin A and it does the job. Thousands of kids have taken it with good results."

Patronizing asshole. Why didn't he answer the question? Was it safe? But really, vitamin A? Sounds pretty harmless. So Chris started taking what sounded like a miracle drug immediately and lo and behold, half a year later the acne had completely disappeared. Gone! We were ecstatic. He was eighteen, in his final year of high school.

And then tragedy hit the family. His father was diagnosed with terminal cancer and admitted to hospital. Day after day, Chris and his sisters and I sat by his bedside, read, made plans, cried and laughed. Every night when we got home I told the kids to wash their hands in warm soapy water because you could never tell what you'd pick up from the hospital, could you?

The day his father died, Chris was curled up on a couch in the waiting room, saying he had a terrible stomach ache. He said the pain felt like a hot nail being driven right though his body. At first I thought he was suffering with grief, but the problem persisted for several days so I dragged myself to the drugstore and bought him antacids. They didn't help. Finally, off to the doctor he went just after his nineteenth birthday. She thought he had an infection of Helicobacter pylori, a bacteria that causes duodenal ulcers. He was given a round of antibiotics. They didn't work. He was given another round. The stomach ache went away for about a month and then he had bouts of bloody diarrhea off and on for the next year. Fools that we were, we thought it was just hemorrhoids.

The next summer he was hired as a wilderness guide for a children's summer camp. He spent two months drinking lake water that had been sterilized with water purification chemicals. On his days off, he and his buddies went into the local town and drank copious amounts of beer and ate pizza and hamburgers. By the time he was twenty and in second-year university, he was pooing blood about twenty times a day.

He had to drop out and come home.

I managed to get him a rush appointment with a gas-troenterologist. Within two days Chris had the first of what would become many colonoscopies. He lay, white as a sheet, in the recovery room, with me sitting at his side as we waited for the doctor to give us the results. Chris was terrified he had cancer and was going to die, just like his Dad.

"Ulcerative colitis," said the harried doctor. "It's very serious — we're going to admit him to the hospital today."

I went home and smoked up the Google search bar. What the hell was ulcerative colitis?

He lay in the hospital bed, day after day, getting thinner and weaker while he pooed blood, now about thirty times a day. He was covered in boils. He had deep cankers in his mouth. He could hardly walk, his joints hurt so much. He had a rash. At night he woke up covered in sweats; during the day his fever spiked.

Chris was very, very sick. Would he die? We watched, terrified. We had just witnessed this same sort of decline in his father.

The doctor decided the only thing to do was to cut the diseased portion of intestine out, but apologetically informed us that his hospital couldn't handle the complexity of the surgery.

Cut it out? Don't you need your intestines?

The next thing I knew Chris was being pushed out of the hospital in a wheelchair so that I could drive him up to North York General in Toronto.

The city lights whizzed by as we headed across town. Chris sighed, "Maybe I drank too much in first year at school."

"This isn't your fault, honey," I replied. But was it? He'd partied pretty hard. But so did lots of kids and they weren't in a wheelchair, unable to walk, pooing blood.

When we arrived at the new hospital I parked at the Emergency entrance, found a wheelchair, and hoped against hope that my son still had all his identification cards in his pockets so that he could be admitted. I had been prepared for a bureaucratic nightmare.

"Name please."

"Chris Curtis."

"Insurance Card."

"Here." He dug in his pocket and produced it.

Amazing.

He was quickly wheeled up to his new room.

His new GI specialist showed up beside Chris's bed about an hour later. Under his nametag were the words "Chief of Medicine." Normally this would fill me with reassurance, but no, a wave of dread washed over me. My son was so sick he needed the very best? The Chief? My dread ramped up to fear. This very smart, wiry man with the clear brown eyes was going to give me a verdict on my son's future. Doctors had the power to tell you if you were going to live or die. I was terrified.

"I know Chris's just had a colonoscopy, but I need to

see for myself what's going on." He looked at Chris and said, "Sorry."

Chris rolled his eyes as a drop of perspiration dripped slowly down his temple, like an errant tear. "You gotta be kidding."

The doctor shrugged and whisked out of the room. In his place a starched nurse, her uniform swishing stiffly, entered the room. She plunked a very large disposable container full of a bubbling liquid on the tray beside Chris's bed.

"Drink that," she said.

Chris looked at her defiantly.

"All up." She actually wagged her finger at him.

Then she wagged her finger at *me*. "Make sure he drinks this!" she said. "The doctor needs a clear view."

As soon as she left I said, "Don't worry, honey." I grabbed the huge container of colon prep off the tray and dumped half of it out into the sink in the corner. He was already cleared out, for heaven's sake!

"Thanks Mom," said Chris, his eyes shutting. "I'll drink it later."

That night I sat in my living room and drank too, only it was six beers. Quickly. His sisters, Elizabeth and Jennifer, on the other hand drank nothing at all as they stonily watched television.

Would he die?

Early the next morning I dashed up to the hospital just as Chris was being wheeled on a gurney into a shiny white procedure room. I stood outside as the doors swung shut. Then both the Chief of Surgery *and* the Chief of Medicine marched importantly into the room wearing their green scrubs. I thanked god for public health care as I totalled up the costs of these two doctors and their mega-salaries. Not that I begrudged them what they were earning; believe me, I was thankful for their level of expertise. In that moment I felt so lucky to have access to such a high level of care. What a great country we lived in.

On the other hand, surely calling in the big guns meant my son was desperately ill. Again terror rose in my throat. I swallowed the fear back down, which began a back and forth battle of gulping with every rising wave of nausea. I felt like a lost and starving bird, repeatedly trying to force a large morsel down my gullet. If only I could fly away into a world where my son was well and tormenting his sisters.

I stood nervously outside the double doors of the procedure room, waiting for the verdict. I listened as hard as I could, trying to hear what was going on. My head jerked back from the crack in the door as a doctor yelled, "Holy shit, look at THAT! Man, is that crater deep!" Then various words seeped through the thin opening in the double doors. First I heard "Surgery." Then I heard "Medicine." Then I heard "Surgery." Then I heard "Medicine."

Were they fighting over my son's treatment? This did not instill confidence. I mean, didn't they *know* what to do?

I stood in the sterile hospital hall listening to the doctors' comments through the door, frightened that my son was going to lose his intestines and have to poo into a plastic bag for the rest of his life. Fear curdled in my stomach. I gulped and gulped as the awful knowledge repeatedly rose and fell in my throat.

The Chief of Medicine finally emerged between the swinging doors and ripped off his green surgical mask. He stood in front of me, his brown eyes somber. "It's very serious. His ulcers are extremely deep. We don't want a perforation. That could kill him."

Then Chris was wheeled out on the gurney, semi-sedated and covered in a white sheet that set off his pale skin. Music from Procol Harum's "A Whiter Shade of Pale" bizarrely bubbled up from the depths of my adolescence and filled my head.

The Chief of Surgery flapped by and said ominously, "No point in saving the intestine if the patient dies. People die from this, you know."

Terror coursed through my veins. My son could die? How on earth did he get this sick? I fought against a tide of helpless tears. I would have to be very strong. This was not good. At all.

The Chief of Medicine gently smoothed the sheet on Chris's bed and carefully put down some of the pictures he had taken of Chris's bowel during the colonoscopy. The bright red and inflamed intestines were stark against the bleached white sheets. I gasped. Even though I had never seen a photograph of the inside of an intestine, I knew this wasn't an example of healthy tissue. My stomach flipped over. The doctor wasn't fooling. The bright red gaping wounds were obvious. It was clear that Chris's illness was serious and dangerous.

I looked at him and said, "Can't you do anything? Is this caused by bacteria? Ulcers are usually caused by bacteria. Will antibiotics help? What do you think?"

The doctor avoided my eyes and said he thought that

Chris had Crohn's disease because of the location of the ulcers in his large intestines. He told me that there was no known cure for the disease and that Chris's life would be in constant jeopardy from a disease that, in the end, would probably kill him.

When you receive devastating news, your mind often reacts in unpredictable ways to soften the blow. Today, with this news that my son had a disease that would ruin his life and ultimately kill him, I bizarrely focused on the 'in the end.' A laugh gathered steam in the base of my chest. My son was going to be killed by his bum! In the end by the end. Ha ha ha.

And then a blast of reality permeated through my skull. This was not funny. Not at all.

So then I got angry. "Crohn's, colitis, ulcerative colitis? What is this? Don't you doctors ever agree on anything? Can't I even get a correct diagnosis?" I crossed my arms and frowned at him in my most 'I am an enraged mother and don't fuck with my kid' look.

The doctor looked down the corridor and didn't reply. His fingers played with some fluff on the sheet. He waited.

The news was beginning to sink in. I knew it was very bad. And I knew in my gut it was caused by bacteria. Of course it was. Why didn't the doctor answer me? I had been rude.

"Sorry."

But then I pressed on and asked the question again. I needed answers and I needed them now. The doctor hemmed and hawed. Finally he looked at me. He said that some people believed it was caused by bacteria but there was debate over which one. He said some researchers thought it was caused by an autoimmune disease, where the body attacks itself, but they weren't sure. He admitted he didn't really know what caused these terrible ulcers, but that a combination of antibiotics, steroids, and an autoimmune medication would hopefully work to settle down the inflammation.

Ah, so Chris was going to be given medicine. The Chief of Medicine had won the battle against the Chief of Surgery. Chris was safe from the knife! Hopefully drugs would work. My fear calmed down a notch.

The wheels on Chris's gurney screeched as he was pushed into an elevator. I put my hand on his arm as a tear rolled down his cheek. He had heard every word. I took a deep breath while my heart twisted into a knot. I had to keep myself together. I couldn't collapse, not now. I put my hand over his and kept it very still as we rode up and up. The dark-haired attendant kept his eyes averted upwards and watched the floors tick by. Chris didn't move his hand away.

My poor baby.

The elevator doors finally slid open at the top floor of the hospital and the gurney squeaked over the shiny linoleum into his new room. A nurse came in and hooked him up to bags and bags of various drugs. Steroids, antibiotics. Saline. Remicade, an autoimmune drug.

I watched an air bubble float along one of the tubes with alarm. Would that travel into his brain and kill him? I flicked at it with my finger. I didn't know if this would actually get rid of the bubble, but I had seen someone do it on TV.

The nurse, who had eyes in the back of her head, whipped

around from wiping down a tray and admonished me. "No touching the tubes."

I looked at my son in despair. He had now lost 65 pounds and was literally skin and bones. I tried to pretend it wasn't happening. Elizabeth, Jennifer, and I decorated his room with get-well cards from his friends and drew pictures of intestines so he could visualize his innards healing. We put on an air of almost hysterical happiness.

Everyone he knew was affected by this illness. Elizabeth couldn't sleep. Jennifer couldn't eat. Chris's friends called, crying because he was in such pain and looked so ill. One flew in from Halifax in the middle of her exams — she couldn't focus.

Chris asked me if he had cancer and if he would die. I said of course not in my jolliest voice. But flames of fear fuelled my every action. I couldn't lose two family members in one year.

That night at home I washed out his bloody boxer shorts and called a nutritionist. I knew that Chris would never get well on hospital food. It was so full of chemicals and sugar and fat it would make anyone sick. She gave me a recipe for a soup that someone with ravaged intestines could digest. I was told to boil spinach, Swiss chard, celery, carrots, dill, and cilantro for twenty minutes. Then I was to add a little salt and puree the concoction of vegetables to a fine, thin, dark green consistency.

I used the handheld blender and splattered the toaster with what looked like green snot.

The next day I fed my weakened son this concoction by hand, trying not to drip the bright green watery liquid on the white sheets. He made valiant efforts to swallow the warm brew but after three gulps he sank back down on the pillow.

"C'mon, have some more, it's good for you," I pleaded.

He didn't move. "Nope. No way. You trying to poison me? It tastes like pond scum."

I rejoiced! He was making jokes. He was rebelling! I laughed and laughed. "You are so funny!"

He mumbled into his pillow, "Yeah, I'm going to be a stand-up comedian." He paused for comic effect and looked at me sideways. "As soon as I can stand up."

After just twenty-four hours of the drug combo, Chris was getting better.

While the hospital's Chief of Surgery hovered over Chris's bed with a knife, the Chief of Medicine held firm. No operation. Yet. We waited to see what would happen next. I felt Chris was getting better. There were some good signs. His fever was down. He could stagger around. He was giving me lip.

Ten days later Chris had another colonoscopy. If he wasn't healing, then it would be surgery.

The doctor came into Chris's room after the procedure. What would he say? I held my breath.

"I can see improvement. The drugs are working."

I was so relieved I could feel tears welling up in my eyes. "Thank you doctor for saving Chris's intestine."

The doctor's kind brown eyes smiled back at me; I could tell he was as relieved as I was. As he turned and left the room he tossed, "For now," over his shoulder.

I shook off the ominous words and kept myself busy by tidying Chris's bedside table yet again. How many straws did one really need? And where was his phone?

Chris kept himself occupied by planning businesses. For a week he was hooked on Crematoriums as being, as he put it, the hot spot of the future. He designed ovens and trucks, letterhead and logos. He talked about refrigeration and corpse decomposition and the consistency of ash mixed with bones.

So disgusting.

But I knew he was dealing with his illness and his father's death. I had to admire his spunk.

For a month Chris lay in the hospital bed and did what he was told, which was to keep a record of his stools; what they looked like, how frequent they were, and what his pain level was. For the first week he wrote "Spaghetti sauce" about thirty times a day. This moved into "Wormies" twenty times a day, then "Hot dogs" ten times a day, and then finally, a month later he was writing, "Tall, dark and handsome" just once a day. Chris was discharged from the hospital with prescriptions in hand for antibiotics and steroids and infusions of Remicade, the biological agent for autoimmune diseases.

When he got home the first thing he did was look in the mirror. I heard a despairing wail from the bathroom. There had been no mirrors in the hospital and he was distraught at what had happened to his body. Kids his age were buff, pumping their muscles, impressing the girls. His body had been eaten away by the disease, whatever it was, and he needed to do some repair work.

I was in awe of his drive. Chris got a gym membership and started to rebuild his body. He still had trouble walking so I bought him an old banger of a car so he could get to the gym. He went back to school. He had fun with his buddies. He took his medication. He was on Flagyl, Ciproflaxin, Prednisone and Remicade.

The Remicade really frightened me. It was touted as an autoimmune drug, or, in other words, a drug that suppressed the immune system. This meant that Chris wouldn't be able to fight off infection. Before each infusion we were called by the pharmacy that was dispensing the drug: did Chris have a fever? A cold? Any flu signs? If he was well, he could then go to his appointment and sit in a chair while a biological agent that tampered with his very marrow dripped into his veins. He went off to a Remicade clinic every eight weeks and chatted with other kids who had Crohn's. Beside each chair hung a bag of Remicade, slowly dripping into their arms.

Some of the kids fell asleep while they waited because the antihistamine that was also in the drug bag caused drowsiness. The antihistamine was to prevent allergic reactions to the drug. During one appointment Chris's face got red, a rash appeared all over his body and his throat became itchy.

"Mom? Mom?" His eyes were wide with fright.

I blasted out of my chair, adrenalin pumping, and screamed, "NURSE!"

She bustled over, calmed us both down, and hooked him up immediately to a bag of steroids to combat the anaphylactic reaction he was having. It turned out, ironically, that he wasn't allergic to the Remicade, he was allergic to the antihistamine!

Once the antihistamine had been taken out of the mix he was fine with the infusions, although the nurse gave him extra steroids and slowed down the drip into his arm every time he went to the clinic. He became known as a "Slow Infuser." Great.

I felt I should be grateful that he was receiving this very expensive drug — it cost thousands of dollars for each infusion — virtually for free through a special drug program in the province. But no, it frightened me. What on earth were the long-term side effects?

Cancer? No one knew.

About six months went by. I spent the time watching him like a hawk while trying to be jovial and carefree. I didn't want him to know how very worried I was all the time. The doctor had said, "For now." Those words rang in my ears and they haunted me. Eventually Chris came off the antibiotics and the steroids although he still went to the Remicade clinic. A few months later the inevitable happened. He got a canker in his mouth. Then a joint hurt. And then he started to bleed again. Again he dropped out of school. Again he lay in bed. Christmas was coming and again he wouldn't be able to snowboard. Or walk.

Back on the antibiotics and Prednisone he went.

So much for the Chief of Medicine. His plan didn't work so great the first time. Clearly the mainstream medical profession was not going to be able to help my son. Where would I have to go to find a cure for this awful disease? Surely it was an infection. Surely it was just bacteria that caused it. Then why couldn't antibiotics cure it?

I felt so desperate. I wanted him *better*. Where were there some answers on how to get him well? We could magnify DNA and take it apart like the spine of a huge dinosaur, we could see each other while talking on the phone, we could accelerate from zero to sixty in seconds, we could even get caramel into a pocket of chocolate. Why couldn't we get my son better? What would I have to do? I knew Chris had the best of the best doctors. Their training was in the best of the best places. We were in a major city with the best hospitals in the country. But, it seemed, the best wasn't going to do the job.

I asked around to all my friends. *Who do you know? Who helped you with odd health things? Who is intelligent and can figure things out?* Finally the name of a woman emerged from three different sources, a general practitioner who repeatedly got in trouble with the College of Physicians and Surgeons because of her willingness to go where other doctors wouldn't. She ventured out of the mainstream. She had a reputation for being open-minded and willing to try alternative treatments, to be creative, to manipulate mainstream knowledge into success. My kind of woman.

I nervously phoned and was told I had to fax my son's story to her. I had to mention how I had heard of her. I had to prove I was open to her way of doing things. And then we got to see her. A file was opened on my son and a new journey began.

This unassuming, conservatively dressed and soft-spoken woman was a quiet warrior against illness. She recommended that Chris go on the Specific Carbohydrate Diet as outlined in a book called *Breaking the Vicious Cycle* by Elaine Gottschall. She pulled a copy off her bookshelf and showed it to us.

Off I trotted to buy it.

I stood in the bookstore and flipped through the pages. Holy smokes, this looked hard. Recipes and long explanations. I knew the next little while was not going to be fun and games. The diet demanded that Chris eat no chemicals in his food and no regular starchy carbohydrates. Good luck with that, I thought as a bag of his favourite kind of potato chips flashed across my mind.

I bought the book and followed it like a bible.

For months and months my son ate differently than every other kid we knew. Most carbohydrates were off the list of foods he could put in his mouth. No bread. No potatoes. No sugar. No pasta. I found a source for almond flour and followed the recipe for baking bread. Hard as a lump of cement, it was barely edible. I sliced and toasted it, pretending that made it better. He could have honey, so I made him candy with honey as the base. I made him French fries out of shredded carrots fried to a crisp in olive oil. When I put them in front of him he said, "Nice try."

The diet demanded that he also have absolutely no chemicals in his diet. No food colouring. No preservatives. Nothing processed. I made him ketchup out of tomato juice. I made him mayonnaise in a blender. I threw out my spice mixtures.

Did it help?

I would have to say it did, up to a point. The symptoms of the disease were somewhat controlled, but not completely. His reaction to this diet convinced me his disease was indeed caused by bacteria and it made sense to me that he was somewhat better because bacteria feeds on carbohydrates. If you limit the carbohydrates that go into your mouth, then the bacteria have nothing to eat and don't multiply. The disease is controlled.

But where the diet really helped was in calming Chris down. He became a very different young man! We had always joked that he was ADD, but on this diet I could see that he had definitely been affected by chemicals in his food. He was so calm! Although this was a great side effect of the diet, there was still something very wrong. My son was still pooing blood. We both knew this wasn't a good thing. Back to the lovely alternative doctor we went.

She tilted back on her chair, thought for a few minutes and then told us about a female patient of hers whose baby son had been diagnosed with Crohn's. She'd been in contact with a doctor in Australia, a Dr. Borody, who was head of the Centre for Digestive Diseases in Sydney. Apparently this doctor believed that Crohn's disease was caused by a bacteria called mycobacterium avium sub-species paratuberculosis, or MAP, and that a combination of four different antibiotics would treat it. The baby had done well with the antibiotics given to him by this doctor.

Eureka! A doctor who was on the same page as I was! All along I had thought the disease was caused by a bacteria and here was the confirmation I needed. I emailed this poor mother, who had obviously suffered a lot, and asked if she could help me.

She called me back the next day and I recognized instantly that knowing this woman would change the isolation I was feeling in my life. She understood my fear, my hopes, my worries. We met for lunch and yakked for hours. She told me about finding blood in her baby son's diaper and I nearly cried because of what she had been through. She told me how Dr. Borody's anti-MAP regimen had worked for her baby, who was now seven. This lovely mother gave me much. She gave me hope that Chris would feel better. She gave me Dr. Borody's email address. She gave me a hug.

I wept with hope and despair as I drafted the Australian doctor an email. I outlined the history of Chris's disease as carefully as I could. I described the medications he'd been on. I listed his symptoms. Would he help my son? I had lost faith in the medical profession but maybe, just maybe, this doctor would be able to help. I put in my contact information and pressed send, hoping for the best.

I actually put my hands together and prayed.

2.
HOPE

I WAS DRIVING through the bush in Northern Ontario when my cell phone rang. Who could that be? Not one of my kids — they were in the car with me. I dug one-handed in my purse for the phone, pressed talk with my thumb and heard a caller with a somewhat British accent ask me if I were Sky Curtis. Who was calling me? And then he announced he was Dr. Borody from the Centre for Digestive diseases in Sydney, Australia. Oh my! It was an *Australian* accent! I nearly dropped the phone. I was flabbergasted. Not only was this extremely busy and famous man calling me personally, he was calling from thousands of miles away to me in the middle of the Canadian Shield! It boggled my mind how small the world had become. I sputtered a polite remark thanking him for his call and then he asked to speak with Chris.

I excitedly handed the phone over to my son, whispering over the hum of the motor, "It's Dr. Borody, the guy I told you about in Australia. I can't believe it!"

"Hiya," snorted Chris.

I whipped my head toward him and frowned my smarten-up look.

I eavesdropped the call unabashedly and knew from

what I was hearing that Dr. Borody was telling my son all about medications and the bacteria they attacked. My clues were Chris saying "MAP" about twenty times. He sounded like a barking dog with a mouthful of marbles. MAP MAP MAP. As the call was winding down Chris handed the phone over to me. "He wants to talk to you."

I pulled the car over and took the phone. A mosquito buzzed around my ear. My three kids fidgeted. The dog panted dog breath over my shoulder. And I was talking to a very famous man who could save my son.

"I've explained to Chris that he needs to send me his chart with the diagnosis and colonoscopy report and I've also described to him the antibiotics I think he needs to combat the MAP bacteria. He probably caught it from diseased cattle. Hamburger. I'll write prescriptions and the drugs will be sent from our pharmacy here. You can pay for them with a VISA card."

"But how will I pay *you*?"

"Don't worry about it."

Don't worry about it? This famous doctor was going to help me, for free? I couldn't believe it. I had absolutely no money. I was still reeling with grief from the death of my husband and traumatized by my son's illness. No way could I work. And yet, I would have sold my house if it meant my son would get treatment. I nearly cried with gratitude and tried to keep my voice from wobbling as I said, "Thank you so much for helping us. It's been terrible." A choke escaped my lips and I swallowed back the tears.

Dr. Borody said, "That's my job. That's what I am supposed to do. He'll get better."

Imagine that. Such kindness. Such generosity. Just like that my despair turned into hope.

After organizing my son's medical chart to be faxed to Australia, Chris then received in the mail a bunch of antibiotics that would make him better. We opened the bubbled wrapped bottles with anticipation and doled out the tablets into a pill organizer. He learned how to swallow six or seven pills at a time. And he got better! Within two weeks my son was completely well on Rifabutin, Cipro-Flaxin, Flagyl, and Clarithromycin, all drugs that target the MAP bacteria, a relative of the same bacteria which causes tuberculosis. He also continued on the Remicade infusions every eight weeks.

There were some side effects from the medication, but nothing like I had expected. His skin took on a tanned look from the medications. He left a yellowish outline on his sheets where he slept. He was on so many pills a day that he had to take a drug to settle his stomach. But that was the extent of the effects. So, Chris's life returned to normal. He started back at school, again, for the winter term. Found himself a nice girlfriend. Got a job. We were overjoyed.

A whole year went by without incident. But then one day he complained about a mouth canker. A boil showed up on his leg. His ankle hurt when he walked. Finally he announced he didn't feel well. And then the bloody diarrhea began. The snow was beginning to fall and, yet again, it looked like Chris wouldn't be playing hockey or snowboarding. Fear flooded my body. Would he lose his intestine this time? We were slowly running out of options.

I leaned on my friends for support. One of them smugly

informed me that Chris needed to deal with his grief of losing his father or else he would never get well. I was livid. First of all, he had a therapist. Secondly, he had an *infection*!

Back to his local specialist, the Chief of Medicine, we went.

"It's been awhile since I've seen you Chris," he said as he flipped through a chart. "Yes, over a year and I think it's time to do another colonoscopy. I need to see what's going on now."

Chris shrugged. "Yahoo."

The doctor smiled as he wrote down a date for a colonoscopy and handed Chris the preparation directions. As we left the hospital Chris tossed them into a garbage bin. I raised an eyebrow at him.

"I got this one down pat, Mom."

Three weeks later Chris was being wheeled out of the same procedure room where he'd been in what seemed like just yesterday, but it was over a year ago. The doctor followed him out and said, "It's bad. In the meantime, I'll write you some prescriptions."

What did he mean, 'In the meantime?' Before what?

With prescriptions in hand, Chris and I drove home from the hospital. Now twenty-three years old, his education in shambles and his self-esteem falling through the floor, he sat quietly beside me. My heart went out to him. His future looked so bleak. "What's up, chum?"

"They think I can't hear them because they've given me drugs. But I know what they said." Chris hiccupped.

"What did they say?"

"That surgeon guy said that I was heading for surgery. Soon." Chris turned his head to hide his hand as he wiped away a tear. "I can't have a bag, Mom."

"Did you say anything back? Could you talk?"

"Yeah. I said, 'NO FUCKING WAY.'"

"You swore? At the Chief of Surgery?"

"Yeah, wouldn't you?"

I had to admire his spirit.

With a heavy heart I called Dr. Borody to let him know the anti-MAP medications had stopped working. That surgery was on the horizon. It was serious.

He was so calm and said, "Sometimes this happens. Some patients stop responding to the medication after about a year. But, I have had success with another treatment, called fecal infusions. It is very extreme and you may not want to do it, but fecal bacteriotherapy may make your son well."

I wasn't keen on that word, 'may.' And 'fecal' didn't fill me with glee either. I knew what it meant. I had an English degree. It meant poo.

Dr. Borody explained that a compromised intestine is vulnerable to an overgrowth of bad bacteria, an infection, which normally would be kept in check by good healthy bacteria. Good healthy bacteria, human probiotics, or in other words, poo, could be used to treat the infection causing Crohn's disease.

"I've had some success by mixing a donor's healthy stool in a sterile saline solution and giving a person with Crohn's/colitis an enema with the mixture. The good bacteria crowds out the bad bacteria and the bowel is put back into balance."

So, I thought, let me get this straight. The good, no, the very famous Dr. Borody was suggesting that I shove shit up my son's ass? I mean, let's call a spade a spade here.

I hemmed and hawed and finally said, "I'll think about it."

After I hung up the phone I shook my head and thought, great, snake oil. Just what we need.

But what were my options for my son? A lifetime of dangerous drugs? Surgery and then more surgery. A colostomy bag? Constant pain? Blood loss? The embarrassment of always needing a bathroom? Would he be able to have a family? Play with his kids? Work? Hell, would he even be able to go back to school? I was so desperate to alleviate his constant suffering.

But poo up his bum? Could I even begin to think about doing *that*? It was so disgusting. It was so weird. It was so, well, just so UGH. But, it made sense. And Dr. Borody was smart. He was kind. But he had also said, "*some* success."

I decided some research was in order and Googled everything I could on the subject. Fecal bacteriotherapy. Human probiotic infusions. Fecal transplants. There was tons of stuff written about this treatment going all the way back to the 1980s. One of my friends told me that vets have been shoving poo up animals' bums for years to get them better from diarrhea.

In short, it wasn't the snake oil I thought it was.

I did even more research. Why were some intestines more susceptible to bowel infections than others? Did I believe in autoimmune diseases? Was that just hogwash invented by doctors who were desperate to explain things?

How did it happen that my son got so sick? Was it the Accutane? The water purification tablets from his canoe trips in the north? The antibiotics? His teenage diet of beer and hamburgers? Why was Crohn's disease on the rise? Who was doing what research? What was new and innovative?

I Googled everything I could find for hours and hours. For some reason that had nothing to do with what I was reading on my computer screen, I began to believe that some people who live in our civilized world are more prone to infection than others. I scrolled down a site about genetic predisposition. Then I thought, so what? Sure, they might be genetically predisposed for the infection, but they wouldn't have become infected unless the conditions in their bowel were just right. After just a little more research, I came to the conclusion that I was right.

A healthy human intestine is packed full with thousands and thousands of species and subspecies of bacteria. I couldn't believe how many. It was disgusting. I put my hand on my stomach as I read about this, convincing myself that I felt the little germs moving. My belly was a zoo. These bacteria all work together in a flora system that keeps our bodies ticking along in a healthy way. But sometimes the bacteria get out of whack and the flora system goes off kilter. We become ripe for infection. Then we can get very, very sick.

How does it happen that our flora systems get off balance?

I read a few articles about the rampant use of antibiotics. I agreed with the articles that said their overuse in our society was one of the main reasons why our flora systems become unbalanced. Almost every person in the western world has been prescribed an antibiotic or other drugs, like Accutane, which wipe out bacteria. These drugs certainly get rid of bacteria which cause infections, pain and even death, but they also kill off the bacteria that promote health. Good bacteria can become depleted because of the use of these drugs, leaving a flora system lopsided and ripe for bad bacteria to take over.

I thought about how we actually live in our civilized society, about our priorities. We are constantly washing ourselves and everything around us. Not so much my house, but, in general. I decided another main reason why a flora system becomes unbalanced was western society's preoccupation with cleanliness. Antiseptic cleansers are used zealously in our kitchens and bathrooms, killing all bacteria in sight. Hand sanitizers are sold by the dozens. They are placed in public places, even by bank machines! Antibacterial soaps and sprays abound in our bathrooms. We rinse our mouths with them. Companies feed upon our fears of getting sick by calling all bacteria 'germs.' In advertisements, these germs are magnified and demonized, often as grotesque cartoon characters that attack people. We are told that if our kitchens are not spotless and gleaming we will certainly get sick. All antibacterial cleansers, just like antibiotics, kill off bacteria that can make us ill, but they also destroy good bacteria that keep our flora systems in harmony.

And I wondered if the food we eat contributed to the problem. I kept an eye open at the grocery store. Shopping carts were filled with boxes of processed food. This didn't seem to be real food at all — there were no vegetables or fruits in sight. Did this cause our flora systems to become shaky? We have become a processed food society. Many of us buy modified food hundreds of times a week, either at fast food outlets or from packages bought at a supermarket. There is a massive industry that sells us convenient food products that have been prepared, en masse, in someone else's kitchen. The main ingredients, whether meat, vegetables, or oils, are mass produced with abundant use of antibiotics, hormones, and pesticides. This 'food' is packed full of colour dyes, chemicals, fat, salt, sugar, and, last but not least, the bacteria from a stranger's kitchen. A flora system, which counts upon us to eat the food it needs to sustain itself, is assaulted, starved, and compromised. I came to another conclusion: our eating habits can also upset our flora system.

A person's flora system can only take so much pounding before it begins to topple. The flora system in a person who eats pure organic unprocessed food but who has been treated with antibiotics twenty times for ear infections is very assaulted. The flora system in a person who has never had antibiotics but eats a fast food hamburger four times a week, repeatedly exposing themselves to diseased cattle and the bad germs that can grow in all sorts of fast food outlets, is being blitzed. The flora system in a person who has never had antibiotics, eats food as pure as the driven snow, but who lives in an antiseptic bubble that has been polished daily with antibacterial products is being ambushed.

It's no wonder bowel infections are on the rise. Almost everyone knows someone with ulcerative colitis and/or Crohn's disease.

When the good, healthy flora system in our intestines becomes too wobbly, the stage is set for a successful invasion of bad bacteria. We get terrible infections. But when our system is active and in a busy balance digesting the unprocessed foods we should be eating, there is no opportunity for bad bacteria to move in and take over. Those germs are immediately crowded out and dealt with by a healthy system.

I read that scientists and doctors around the world are discovering evidence that many of the bowel diseases we now suffer from are caused by an infection of bad bacteria. This evidence has taken years and years to surface because the bowel is convoluted and very, very long. Bacteria can hide in all the nooks and crevasses of a bowel. It has been extremely difficult to identify the bacteria and even to find it. Research is being done to develop accurate tests to help identify which specific bacteria cause which diseases. Once the bacteria is accurately identified, doctors will be able to develop and prescribe the correct antibiotic, which targets that particular bacteria.

But wait! What's wrong with this picture? The antibiotic does not just target the culprit bacteria, it also destroys other bacteria in a person's intestines, thus leaving the bowel open to an unbalanced flora situation. This, of course, is one of the reasons the infection takes hold in the first place. A person's infection may be dealt with, but you can count on a new infection taking root in a year or two. Guaranteed. So, what are the alternatives?

Doctors are under huge pressure to prescribe drugs to treat diseases. Drug companies circle around them, offering free samples and shiny pamphlets on drugs that treat these infections. Antibiotics, anti-inflammatory drugs, immune suppressants, pain inhibiters, you name it, they want to sell it and make a ton of money. The drug industry is very interested in sustaining itself by selling drugs. These companies employ thousands and thousands of people and any threats to it are immediately squashed.

In the meantime, the percentage of people who suffer from bowel diseases is increasing rapidly because of antibiotics, extreme cleanliness, and processed foods. People stream in and out of doctors' offices suffering from diarrhea, bloating, gas, cramps, weight loss, pain, bleeding, and so on, including terrible secondary offshoots of these symptoms such as boils, rashes, sore joints, and non-functioning livers. A huge industry is growing because there are more and more people who are in pain, fading away, and often dying from bowel diseases. Thus, the question arises, if antibiotics actually help create an environment for infection to exist, how do we treat bowel diseases caused by infection?

Antibiotics are 'anti' life, while probiotics are 'pro' life. Antibiotics kill off bacteria, whereas probiotics are full of bacteria. After a person is prescribed antibiotics, many members of the medical profession tell that person to eat yogurt, or take a probiotic purchased from a health food store to replace some of the good bacteria that has been killed off by the antibiotic. People who suffer from various bowel ailments are almost always much improved by taking over the counter probiotics.

All around the world research is being done to assess the effectiveness of probiotics in treating various bowel diseases, including Crohn's and ulcerative colitis. This is no easy task. Our bowels are full of hundreds and hundreds of bacteria and it is very difficult, if not impossible, for the pharmaceutical industry to mimic this complicated healthy environment. Many of the bacteria aren't even identified.

It would be even more difficult to ascertain which bacteria were out of balance in any given person because each person's body is unique. What is off kilter for one person might be perfect for another. How would anyone be able to assess the situation, no less correct a flora system that is out of whack and rife with a single bacteria that has multiplied, causing a terrible infection, or in other words, an over-growth of one bacteria?

I read about epidemics in hospitals of superbugs. When there is an outbreak of intestinal bacteria such as C. difficile or lysteria, some people die and some do not. Some get a simple stomach ache for a night and some have diarrhea for years. This is all due to the health of the sick person's flora system. Some people have healthy systems, and some simply do not for a variety of reasons, but mainly because of antibiotics. A person with a flora system that is unbalanced is at high risk for developing a bowel disease.

So, at the end of all this research, I had to ask myself the one most important question: How does one create a well-balanced flora system that will crowd out the bad bacterial growth? I didn't much like the answer.

With poo.

Dr. Borody was on to something. I was becoming convinced that fecal bacteriotherapy might just work. It made so much sense.

Most people think of poo as disgusting. That's because it is. It stinks. We are all taught from a very young age that our stool is full of germs. It is. It is full of the bacteria that flourishes in our systems.

Yet, poo is the very best probiotic known to man. It's free. It's readily available. It's completely natural. And, apparently, it works.

In my research I read how C. difficle, a terrible infection that kills vulnerable people, is now being treated with fecal bacteriotherapy, a probiotic full of good bacteria, namely, poo. There is a large study underway right now at Toronto General Hospital assessing the effectiveness of fecal enemas in treating this fatal bacteria. Doctors all over the world know that this treatment is effective, but being doctors, they have to have the scientific evidence. They also have to get over their personal aversions, their "ick factor." More than this though, they have to have approval from their ruling bodies to do fecal infusions or else risk losing their licences to practice medicine.

A person who is dying from a C. difficle infection will do anything to live. Those who are lucky will be treated with human probiotic infusions. This is a complicated way of saying that a person who is suffering from C. difficile is getting poo from a healthy person put into their digestive system. Just one treatment can save a person's life. Dr. Borody has a very high success rate, as do Canadian doctors. The ethical questions are, I'm sure, enormous, but not as enormous as the loss of a life if one doesn't get a fecal infusion.

But the resistance to this treatment is huge. Pharmaceutical companies don't make a penny from it so they slam it. The medical profession is so pharmaceutically based they are very wary of a natural treatment. People in general are disgusted by it. But those who are very sick, some even close to death, will do anything to get better. They think nothing of putting healthy poo up their bums. To them the choice is simple: to die or to live, to lose their bowel and defecate into a bag for the rest of their life, or to get better and keep their intestine. To be permanently crippled with joint pain or to walk and run. To these people, it's a no-brainer.

In the meantime Chris had an appointment with the Chief of Medicine.

"It's a serious situation," he said as we both sat tensely in front of him.

"What do you think about fecal transplants?" I asked. "Dr. Borody thinks they might help."

"They like that in Australia."

"Yes, but, what do *you* think?" I needed to know because I didn't want Chris to lose his home doctor if the transplants didn't work. Also, if anything went wrong, then we would need help. Could they go wrong?

"Well, they won't harm him," said the doctor.

I was much encouraged by this answer. He could have simply said, "They're hogwash!"

Later Chris and I talked about Dr. Borody's suggestion of trying fecal transplants. We looked at the very few other options available to help Chris and we agreed: it was worth a try. Once we got that far we got down to the nitty-gritty of the thing. Who would be the donor?

"I think you should do it, Mom. You are by far the healthiest person in the family. Plus you go every day."

Jennifer said, "Not me, I just go all the time. That can't be right."

I replied, "It's all the legumes you eat, being a vegetarian."

Elizabeth said, "I think it should be you Mom, you are so healthy."

And so it was decided. I would be the donor. My first thought was, "Would I have to stop drinking?" But what I said out loud was, "Thanks honey, for the vote of confidence. I am pretty healthy. And reliable."

I called Dr. Borody back.

"We've talked about it and have decided to try it out. We'll give it a go."

Dr. Borody laughed at my inadvertent joke. So did I.

"I'm going to be the donor. Am I allowed to drink?"

"Sure! No worries."

Love those Australians.

"I'll get one of my staff to send you an information package on how to do home infusions. In this package there are instructions on diet and medications, plus a shopping list of the various items you will need to do the infusions. It will also contain a list of the blood and stool tests you need to do to ensure that you are a healthy donor."

I now had a mission that made sense to me. I believed in it. My son was going to have fecal infusions! My healthy bacteria was going to crowd out his bad bacteria. He would get well. I didn't know if I was excited or disgusted. But finally I had a legitimate reason to give my son shit!

3.
INSTRUCTIONS

THE INSTRUCTIONS for home transplants arrived in my email account the next day from Dr. Borody's Centre for Digestive Diseases in Australia. I downloaded everything he sent me and held the sheets of paper in my hand as if I were holding the Holy Grail. Here were the instructions on how to get my son well! Of course they would work! It was all good. I was filled with hope.

I sat at my desk with the pages in front of me and began to read. In general, it was hard for me to concentrate during that time because I always had half an ear listening for Chris. I was very aware of every trip he made to the bathroom. I'd hear him slowly make his way along the hall, his feet shuffling on the carpet. I'd worry about him falling down in the bathroom and listen for sounds of him fainting. I'd call out to him, "Are you dizzy, honey? Get off the toilet slowly and take deep breaths." I knew that every time he stood up he saw black. I couldn't relax until I heard the toilet flush, his feet drag back down the hall and back up the stairs. Then I could focus on whatever I was doing until the next time he had to go, just minutes later.

While I was listening for sounds of movement in the house I read the information about diet for both the donor and the recipient. I looked at this carefully. No processed food for either of us. No chemicals. No foods that commonly cause food poisoning, like deli meats and shellfish. I was to eat a high carbohydrate and high fibre diet. Before the infusions Chris was to have a low carbohydrate, low fibre diet. After the infusions began, he would need a high carbohydrate diet.

All of this made sense to me. Putting chemicals into the body of a person with open ulcers seemed a sure bet for causing cancer. Eating food that had a reputation for going rotten easily seemed a folly if you were already dealing with intestinal difficulties. I would need lots of carbohydrates because they provided the sugars that bacteria feed on and it would be a good thing for me to have active bacteria. Plus, as a donor, I would need lots of fibre to make sure I went to the bathroom every day, without fail.

Chris on the other hand certainly didn't need help with going to the bathroom or with having active bacteria so it made sense that he needed, up until the infusions, a low carbohydrate diet with very little fibre. Once the infusions began he would have to change his diet to a high carbohydrate one in order to feed the new bacteria in his system. He'd been watching his carbohydrates for ages so this was nothing new. He'd kill for a potato chip.

I ran upstairs to tell him the good news. "You can eat all the carbohydrates you want once we begin the infusions! Pasta! Cereal! Rice!"

He looked at me from under his covers as if I were missing the point.

"Mom-m-m-m. French fries. Pop. Hamburgers. Pizza. Ice cream."

"It's been hard, hasn't it?"

"When can I start eating junk food again?"

"I haven't finished reading the instructions yet, but as soon as we start the infusions I'll get you some treats. But that's all they are, you have to eat well from now on."

I didn't have the heart to tell him that hamburger was probably out of the question for the rest of his life. There was now very strong evidence that the MAP bacteria came from diseased cattle.

I returned to my office and read the directions for the medications Chris would need before the first transplant. It was recommended that he take a cocktail of antibiotics, most of which he'd already been on for the past year. I imagined that this was to get rid of as much of the bad bacteria as possible before the infusions began so that the new bacteria would have a fighting chance to become established. Unfortunately, these antibiotics had stopped working and were no longer keeping the bad bacteria in check. This was why, in fact, I was reading these directions in the first place!

Did it matter that he wasn't taking effective antibiotics? Would the infusions be able to take hold? Were my little bacteria going to be overwhelmed by his bad bacteria? I had no idea. I just had to trust that the infusions would work, regardless of not being able to do this step adequately.

And what about the Remicade? Dr. Borody had said Chris had to stop taking the Remicade infusions. Immune suppressants were a no-no. As much as I believed that Remicade did absolutely nothing in controlling Chris's symptoms and as much as I didn't believe in autoimmune hocus pocus, rightly or wrongly, and as much as I abhorred the idea of all those chemicals going into his body, it still frightened me to take him off it. I had been led to believe that once a person was off Remicade, the chances of the drug being effective on a restart-up were close to nil. Ironically the body built up an immunity to the drug. This meant that if the fecal infusions didn't work, then Remicade would no longer be a treatment option.

And then I thought, so what? It wasn't working anyway. Had it ever worked? Maybe a bit, for a month or two. I laughed at my worries and kept on reading. He was to stop all antibiotics the day before the first infusion. In the past they had certainly been a lifeline, but no longer. They didn't work! I was so relieved that Chris would be free of all these chemicals. If the infusions didn't work, then maybe the break from the antibiotics would allow them to be effective again.

"Hey Chris," I yelled up the stairs, "No more Remicade or pills."

I listened. No answer. Was he okay? I pushed my chair away from my desk and climbed up the stairs to check on him, my heart thumping. I had my cell phone with me in case I had to call 911. I lived in a state of constant fear that I would find him either passed out or dead.

I opened his bedroom door, hand shaking, only to see he was sound asleep. He looked like an angel, finally getting some small respite from the pain. I tiptoed down the stairs. That poor boy never got a chance to sleep longer than forty minutes because he had to keep getting up to go to the bathroom and I sure wasn't going to wake him up now.

When I got back to my desk I read over the blood and stool tests. They made me feel slightly nauseous. Couldn't we just skip this part? Was it important that I be tested as a donor? And then I sat up straight. Of course I had to take the tests. It had to be determined that I was a healthy donor. Tests take time. We didn't have time. I had to take them NOW. I was in a rush. Christmas was coming and the holiday schedule would interrupt the lab results from coming back in a timely fashion if I didn't get my samples in to the lab very soon.

Chris was so sick, the last thing I wanted was to delay the infusions by even a day if it could be helped. A week more in his condition would probably mean surgery. Right then I made a rush appointment to see our alternative doctor for a requisition form for the tests and dashed to her office. Afterwards I immediately went to the lab and picked up the right vials for the poo tests. I made sure the lids screwed on tightly. Wouldn't want any spillage of THAT.

I read the stool test instructions carefully and for the next week I gathered up what I needed for the little vials with a popsicle stick and put my booty into various solutions of various bottles over various days. It wasn't pleasant, but considering what I was going to be doing with it in just a little while, I considered this small potatoes. It was practice. Not a problem.

Once the collection of all those samples was done and I could hand them in to the lab, I had to face the music. While I was at the lab, handing in my vials of doo-doo,

I thought I should probably get the blood tests done as well. For most people this wouldn't be a problem. For me? Big problem. First of all, I hated needles. Secondly, I was terrified of the results.

And so it was that I was sitting in a plastic chair in the lab's small waiting room, with vials of poo at my feet in a plastic shopping bag and sweat dripping down my back. My mind raced. I couldn't believe I was doing this. I was going to get my blood tested. Me! Unbelievable.

For the past ten years my family doctor had urged, no begged, me to get a blood test. She had cited various reasons with her brow furrowed, a scowl turning her lips down. She had admonished me, repeatedly, for a decade. I was irresponsible. I was foolish. I was walking around with malaria. Whatever. For ten years I just rolled my eyes. It wasn't going to happen. I would not get a blood test. I would not have my life blood removed.

I would not find out what was up.

It's not that I was worried about my cholesterol levels. I was a runner plus I had a full tablespoon of cod liver oil every day, not to mention Omega this and that. I kept my joints and arteries oiled. I had no concerns about sexually transmitted diseases. HIV was not on my radar. Believe me, I knew where I had been. Sadly, nowhere. I felt fine, thank you very much.

And that was sort of the problem. I felt really fine. Better than fine. Really, really great. Happy great. Especially at night. I couldn't have felt better. If you catch my drift.

I drank like a fish!

I had avoided a blood test for years, mainly because I was terrified of what it would reveal about my liver. I was a party girl. Every night I liked to drink beer and read a book. Some nights I drank too much. I knew this. I didn't care. It was fun. The family joke was when I died you'd have to beat my liver with a stick to make it lie still.

So, no, I didn't want to get my blood tested. What if the test told me I was going to die of liver disease?

These were my thoughts as I sat in the little waiting room, hungry because I hadn't eaten in twelve or more hours because of one of the tests. I waited for someone who I hoped was a well-trained technician to jab me and suck out my blood. I dreamed fondly of little tiny mosquitoes.

I had taken special care with my clothing that morning. I tried to look extra nice so I'd be treated with respect. Gently. Carefully. I wore a shirt with sleeves that could roll up easily. I wore a nice scarf. I had on earrings. My nails were filed and clean. The plastic bag containing vials of crap at my feet sort of wrecked the picture of refinement, but I had done the best I could.

The blood test requisition was a list a mile long. They'd need a barrel to contain all the blood they needed from me. At this thought I almost bolted from the waiting room. But, Dr. Borody had given me the list and I knew, in my heart of hearts, that it would be best if I got myself cleared as a healthy donor. Sweat kept dripping down my sides. I needed a drink. I was not a happy camper.

Finally my name was called. I handed in the poo vials to the technician and she plopped them down, unfeelingly I thought, on a metal table. I worried about them getting lost and tossed them a fitful glance as I walked past and followed her down the white tiled hallway. I eyed the rubber hose she was carrying with fear. I knew what that was for. She was going to wrap it around my arm! And then steal my blood!

The sanitary hall tilted as my heels clacked on the shiny tiles. Little black dots danced across my vision. She led me to a chair attached to an arm rest and I fell thankfully into it. Her hands were warm as she stretched out my arm and tied it up with the hose. She told me to open and close my fist.

I wanted to bop her one. But she had the needle.

She lined up eight vials in front of her on a little platform thing beside my arm. EIGHT. I'd be dead if they took that much blood from me. I tried not to look at them. I had a fantasy of my body deflating like a spent balloon. My eyesight clouded and cleared and clouded again. My head reeled.

Suddenly the vampire told me to stop clenching my fist and to blow out suddenly. I wasn't fooled by her infantile diversion tactic. I could feel the jab. And then it started, the sucking noise of my blood being drawn into the vials. It went on and on forever. I thought I would throw up. I thought I would die. I thought I would faint. And then it was over. She pressed a cotton ball onto what was surely a gaping wound and told me to hold it.

"There, all done," she said and gave me a reassuring pat. "You did very well. What kind of bandaid do you want? Little Bo Peep or Superman?"

I pathetically whispered, "Superman," and watched as she put a bandaid on the tiny red dot where the needle had been.

She gathered up the maroon-filled vials and labelled them all with my name. "There, you're fine to go. The result will be here in about a week. You can call your doctor for them."

The results? YIKES. I needed a drink. No, I didn't. My liver had better be fine. I scurried away and finally made it back to my car, where I panted and gripped the steering wheel. I had done it! I would find out if I could give a shit. I laughed uncontrollably at my joke. And then I sobered up completely. I had to help my son. I *had* to be healthy.

4.
THE SHOPPING LIST

WHILE I WAITED for my blood and stool test results to come back, I decided it would be a productive use of time to get the equipment for the infusions. This forward-looking activity would help confirm my faith that I would be well enough to do infusions. Yes, it was time to get the show on the road. My son needed his first transplant soon and time was of the essence. I had to go shopping.

I hated shopping.

I leafed through the instruction package Dr. Borody had sent me until I found the list of items I needed. Believe me, it was no ordinary list. No Cheerios or socks in sight on a fecal transplant list. The list said:

psyllium husks
disposable enema bags
water-based lubricant
sterile saline solution
toilet hat
latex gloves
blender
spoon

My eyes travelled down the list when I suddenly stopped. Toilet hat? What? I had no idea what a toilet hat was. Dancing cats with canes and top hats flew across the stage of my mind. Nah, couldn't be. It was probably one of those plastic white containers that hung like an upside down hat off the toilet bowl rim so you could collect your poo. I'd seen one in the hospital when Chris had been there. That's right, I remembered the nurse carrying it off to the lab after he'd gone. They kept checking him for C. difficile. That had not inspired confidence in the cleanliness of the hospital.

But where on earth would I get all these very medical items?

Many women love to shop. They even know where to go for what. If they want to buy jewelry they go to a jewelry store. Me? I wait for the moment to pass. If they want to buy a radio, they go to an electronics store. Me? I get in my car and push a button. *Voilá,* a radio! I am not a shopping kind of gal. I can't stand it. I hate everything about it. The florescent lights, the aisles, the slippery floors, the dust bunnies in the corners. The zealous sales help. And I really hate the change rooms with what are certainly circus mirrors that make you look extra wide.

The first problem, of course, was where to go to get the stuff on my list. You can get almost anything you need at second-hand stores but I wasn't too sure about enema bags. I didn't recall seeing a section called "Bum Notions" at The Salvation Army Thrift Store. No sirree. I had to do some serious shopping.

Secondly, did I really need it all? Could I make do with something from around the house? I had a blender. I had a spoon. Then I thought about it. I was using these things to mix up POO so I could put it into my son's BUM. I banished the thought of double duty for these items quickly. NO NO NO! I needed brand new items that would be used for this job and this job alone. They could not be used for anything else. These items needed to be thrown out at the end of the task. When he was well.

Yeah, right.

No, it had to work. It would. Pray pray pray.

I debated long and hard about the psyllium husks. I'd read an article once about companies that make cake mixes. They discovered after much research that housewives felt guilty if they weren't making a cake from scratch. Just as an aside here, I didn't make up the term "housewives." That was made up by men. Anyway, the companies could easily concoct a cake mix that didn't need anything at all but a cup of water. But, no, a cup of water wasn't enough to assuage the guilt of a woman who had sneakily resorted to a cake mix. So, to get rid of the guilt which might hold her back from buying the product, the cake mix company put recipes on the back of the box that said to add an egg, maybe milk, and some even went as far as requesting a tablespoon of melted butter. The theory was if a woman put some butter in the microwave and zapped it for thirty seconds, she would feel like she was truly baking for her family and the guilt would be gone.

Where did men get these ideas?

So, when I pictured myself making the slop out of poo, I had to ask myself about the necessity of the psyllium husks. Were they really needed? Were they in the recipe, so to speak, to make me feel better about what I was doing? To make me feel as if I were really taking care of this situation? They were hard to find. They were expensive. I called Dr. Borody.

"No, they're good to put in, they give some food for the bacteria to feed on. It makes the healthy bacteria more robust."

Robust? My imagination took off. I pictured a puny little bacteria munching on a husk and then turning into a GI Joe, beating his chest and swimming upstream in my kid's intestines, punching out the bad bacteria and taking over. Okay, I'd buy the psyllium husks. But where would I find them? Probably the health food store. I called, and while I waited for someone to answer I swore I could smell the incense in the air. Yes, they had them. The sales help sounded as if she'd been zenned to death.

Next on the list were disposable enema bags. Where on earth does one find disposable enema bags? Certainly not at a hardware store. I picked up the yellow pages and lazily flipped through it, looking at the various sections: Automotive? Nah. Furnaces? Nope, Lawyers? No way. Pet Stores? Don't think so. Suddenly, floating up from the depths of my memory bank was the image of a friend I had in Grade Twelve. Good ole Vivian. I wonder where she is today. It was the Pet Stores that triggered my memory.

Vivian was an earnest looking girl, just a little overweight with thick glasses and she worked in a drug store that carried some medical supplies, like walkers and bedpans. Not because she needed the money — her parents were rich — but because they wanted her to learn the value of a dollar. Off she went to the drug store every Tuesday and Thursday after school to make her spare cash so she could buy her marijuana without her parents asking where her money went. She had her teenage reply ready: "It's my money and I'll do what I want with it." Vivian knew the value of a dollar all right; ten of the little things would get her a dime bag.

One day while this earnest, slightly stoned girl was dusting shelves in The Health Aid Drug Store, a very old, thin, white haired lady came in and asked my happy, healthy ox of a friend, "Do you have an enema bag?"

Well. Who at the age of sixteen has ever heard of an enema bag? Certainly not Vivian. She stood up from her dusting, towered over the little lady, and said quite loudly — because, as you know, all little old ladies are deaf — "Animal bag? Animal bag? They're sold across the street. At the pet store." Vivian shouted, "PET STORE."

The little old lady went pale. "No, *enema* bag," she quaked. "I need an enema bag."

Vivian took the little old lady by her bony elbow and walked her to the plate glass window at the front of the shop and pointed across the street. She spoke very slowly. "See, over there, that's the pet store. You can find an animal bag there."

Vivian's finger veered slightly to the left as if drawn by a magnet and pointed to the bakery next door to the pet store. She licked her lips. She was always hungry and we know why.

"Enema bag," the little old lady crowed. "I need an enema bag."

By now the pharmacist was aware of the commotion. He strode briskly down the aisle and said, "Here, Mrs. Cruikshank, the enema bags are down here." He bent over and handed her a package of what looked like a hot water bottle with a hose on it.

When Vivian told the story, she could hardly contain herself as she told me how she had read the directions on the package. She was laughing so hard she had to cross her legs tight to stop herself from wetting her pants as she recounted how the package crinkled loudly. It was all so very funny for Vivian but I didn't really get why. That's because I didn't know what an enema bag was. I laughed anyway. And not because I wanted her weed. I didn't smoke. Asthma.

But Vivian knew I was just trying to look cool. Under her thick glasses her eyes suddenly became accusing beach balls. "You don't know what an enema bag is, do you? She was so smug with her now superior knowledge. "It's a bag like a water bottle with a hose on it to shove up your BUM."

I remember being aghast.

But now I knew I needed to find a drug store that sold medical supplies as well. A medical supply place, just like where Vivian used to work. I looked down the list. The next five items, water-based lubricant, sterile saline solution, toilet hat and latex gloves could all be purchased at a medical supply store. I loved one-stop shopping.

But wait a minute. If I was pooing into the toilet hat (oh please) wouldn't my pee get in there as well? How bad was pee? Was it absolutely forbidden in the poo? Again I called Dr. Borody.

"I know you usually use men for donors, and men have this advantage in that they can hang their…." I stopped here, did I say "penis" to Dr. Borody? Oh dear. "Hang their junk away from the toilet hat so they don't get any pee on the...."

"Shit," said Dr. Borody.

"Yes, exactly. But women have this situation where they can't do this. How bad is it to get pee on the shit?"

"You don't want to do that."

"Oh," I said. "How do I prevent this?"

"Be creative."

"Oh."

"You are a very brave woman."

Or crazy, I thought. I hung up. So, no pee in the poo. Maybe I needed to buy a urinal to clamp on over the right hole while the other hole was busy. So to speak. I added urinal to my personal list. I would find one, no doubt, at the medical supply store.

The next item, a blender, could be bought at the hardware store. The last item, a spoon, I surely didn't need to buy. Surely I had an extra spoon that I would never need to use again. I took my list and off I went, shopping. My first stop was the medical supply store.

5.

MEDICAL SUPPLY STORE ADVENTURE

I MARCHED INTO the antiseptic glare of the medical supply store with my head held high. I would not be embarrassed. I would be cool, clear, concise. I would get what I needed to give my son a fecal transplant. I dug through my purse for my list and refreshed my memory: enema bags, water-based lubricant, sterile solution, surgical gloves, a toilet hat and now, newly added, a urinal. My stomach cringed with embarrassment. I straightened my back and calmed myself down. Remember, I said to myself, the staff here deals with bodily functions every day. They won't bat a collective eyelash.

I was descended upon by one of the reasons why I hated shopping, a zealous sales person. She snatched the list out of my hand and paraded towards the far reaches of the store. I limped behind her, my head slightly bowed, cheeks flaming red. So much for my resolve. She screeched to a stop and I nearly banged into her.

"How many enema bags?" She gestured elegantly at a display case as if she were the hostess on some game show. Her prizes sparkled on a shelf. There were hundreds of clear plastic-wrapped enema bags, their transparent hoses maliciously glinting under the fluorescent lights.

How many indeed? Ten? Twenty? Four hundred thousand? My mind was racing.

"How much are they?"

"About $6.00 each."

I picked one up and examined it. She was getting impatient. I think her foot was tapping. But I had to see what they were. I'd never seen an enema bag. My mind whirred. Was it a good deal? Did I have options? Could I get them cheaper elsewhere? Hmm, probably not. I saw a hole in the end of the hose.

"Is this defective? There's a hole." I tried not to think about the hose going you know where.

"That's to bathe the area with the solution."

The area? Well, there's a nice little euphemism for an asshole.

"And is the tip, you know," I choked a bit here, thinking of my poor boy. "Rounded?"

She looked at me as if I were insulting her personally and said arrogantly, "Of course it is. But many people use a water-based lubricant to ease things along."

She was pissing me off. I said snippily, "Yes, it's on my list." I reached over and tapped the list she smugly held in her hand. She clutched it to her chest. A power struggle had just been announced.

"How many?" she challenged.

"Twenty," I replied with a flourish.

She counted out twenty, exactly, and sailed over to the lubricants. "Small or large?" she asked while pointing at the two sizes and speaking as if to a moron.

"Large," I said defiantly.

She put a large tube into the shopping basket that had

somehow miraculously appeared over her left arm. She guarded it with her right arm, the list still clenched in her hand. She was winning the power struggle. Then she, the Attila the Hun of sales help, peered at my list. "Sterile solution? Is it for nasal spray or irrigating wounds?"

She had me there. But then I thought. A little spray wasn't going to do this job. I needed lots and lots I said, "Wounds."

"What size then? Five hundred millilitres or a litre."

How the hell would I know? I'm old. I wasn't brought up with these newfangled measurements. How much is five hundred millilitres?

"How big is a litre?" I asked sheepishly.

She gestured with her hands, a sneer playing at the corners of her mouth. It was about the size of a quart of milk.

God, I hated shopping. "Five hundred millilitres, then."

"How many bottles?"

I could always come back for more. "Five."

The basket sagged towards the right as she lined up five bottles in the bottom. Her arm got those funny white marks where the handle dug into her flesh. Served her right for being so controlling.

She swooped over to the gloves. There were boxes and boxes of them. A whole shelf the length of the store. How would I ever decide? The various sizes and contents danced dizzyingily in front of my eyes.

"Latex?"

I thought about my son and all his allergies. "No, probably not."

She stepped in front of a different bank of boxes. "Powdered?"

I thought of the powder going into the slurry. "No, no powder."

She moved to the right. "What size?"

We both had to wear them. He had big hands and mine were small. "Medium."

"A box of a hundred? Or more?"

"A hundred should do us."

She grabbed a box and flung it into the basket.

I was exhausted. The decisions about gloves alone would qualify me to be the next Prime Minister! My therapist would be so proud of me.

"Us?" She looked at me quizzically, as if I were into some weird sex triangle.

"Toilet hats?" I responded, nonchalantly.

She whisked down the aisle and threw one into the basket before I could even look at it. Was it really what I wanted? Could I poo into it? What were those lines I saw on the inside? Were those measurements? Should I be able to measure the output versus how much food I ate? Was it important? I desperately wanted to grab the basket away from her and look at it. She, the next Minister of Defense, clamped her elbow tightly to her side. No way was I going to get that basket. But on to the last item. Finally, down to the urinal!

She stood in front of what looked like lopsided green vases that smelled of plastic. I guessed that was better than smelling like pee. "Male or female?" she said.

"Pardon?"

"Male or female? Do you need a male urinal or a female urinal?"

How would I know? "Ah, what's the difference?"

She looked at me as if saying "Duh." Then she put down the basket so she could thrust the two different types in front of my nose. I saw my chance. The basket was mine, all mine! I swooped it up, triumphantly. I was now the boss.

"Thanks for all your help, I'll take it from here."

She snorted, turned on her heel, marched down the aisle and disappeared, only to snap up the next customer two aisles away. I was blessedly on my own.

I cautiously put down the basket, looking this way and that. No one was around. Medical supply stores do not have fitting rooms. I needed a fitting room! For what I had to do now, I really needed privacy.

I had to try the urinals on. You would think that because I was a female it would make sense to use a female urinal. However, I was using it for a very different reason than the usual one and perhaps the shape wasn't the most conducive to this particular job, so to speak. Which one would work better? I imagined myself sitting on the toilet, the hat in place, and stuffing a urinal in between my legs to catch any pee. I looked around, saw no one, and quickly stuffed the male one between my legs. Hmm. Then the female. Hmm. I looked up, checking for people. Not a soul. I tilted my head to the side and thought. The female one seemed to work better. No doubt about it. But I had to make sure. I spread my legs and tried it again, for good measure. Then I balanced on one leg and tried to get it clamped on good and tight. I lost my balance a bit, but grabbed onto some shelving to save myself. Yup, it would be fine. I put a female urinal in the basket and lugged the goods to the nearest counter with a cash register. Phew, no one saw that little show.

I was proudly lifting all my pickings out of my basket onto the counter when I just happened to glance up. Right over the pretty little sales girl's blond head was a mounted television screen. On the screen was the aisle I was just in. I could see the green vases all lined up, lopsidedly sitting on the shelf. I saw a customer walk by, pick one up and put it in her basket.

I had trouble breathing. I could hear my blood pounding in my ears. My face was burning up. Sweat was trickling down my back. I lowered my eyes to the cute little sales girl. I knew she had seen me jamming that green urinal between my legs.

Oh god! I cringed. I just hated shopping.

She smiled sweetly. "Find everything you wanted?"

I looked into her innocent blue eyes. They didn't even flicker. Ah good, she hadn't been watching.

"Yes, thanks." I was oh so very blasé.

She took the items out of the basket one by one, scanned them for their prices and then put them into a bag. Then she reached for the last item in the basket, the urinal, and winked at me.

6.

CHOOSING A BLENDER

AFTER A COUPLE OF DAYS' rest from my exhausting shopping adventure in the medical supply store, I braced myself for more purchases. I still needed a few more items on my list: psyllium husks and a blender. I plugged my nose and held my breath as I sailed through the incense at the health food store and found the section for psyllium husks. I grabbed the smallest bag that would still probably last me thirty years, paid, and raced out. One item down, one to go. Off to the hardware store.

I already had a blender; don't get me wrong, my kitchen is certainly well-equipped. But somehow I felt I needed a new one for this particular task alone. Cheap as I am, it seemed a small price to pay. And so I stood in front of a row of shelves stacked with boxes of blenders. Their shiny packages glittered, revealing all their advertised features: their wattages, their tight lids, their dependability, but most of all, their buttons.

There were buttons galore. Buttons for liquefying, buttons for grinding, buttons for cleaning, buttons for crushing ice. Who would've guessed blenders had so many functions? How on earth would I know which blender was the best one for my job? Ha ha. Such a comedian.

What button did I really need? The pulse? The grate? The whip? This was definitely outside my area of expertise. Milkshakes I understood. Soups? A breeze. Blending crap? No experience.

And just how does shit behave in a blender? Is it turbulent? I started to snicker to myself. "Oh grow up," I said out loud. Then I laughed again.

Sometimes life is hilariously bizarre. This was one of those times. I stood in front of the blenders and hummed, "Dum de Dumm Dum." In my head I was really singing "Bum de Bumm Bum," but no one would know. I was trying to look so cool but laughter giddily burst out from inside my chest as I contemplated blending shit.

I knew I was laughing because I was trying to cope with my son's horrible situation. I was worried. I was frightened. I was exhausted. I was very silly. I tried to compose myself and scanned the rows. What, exactly, did I need? First of all it had to be very easy to clean. Very, very easy. It had to be made out of glass so it wouldn't absorb the smell of poo and stink. It had to cope with chunks. I hated to admit that part, but it was true. Chunks could be a problem.

I remembered once trying to make asparagus soup by blending the tough ends. Try as I might with spatulas and double blending, it just didn't work out for me. The soup was full of tough chunks. And since then, well, of course I've had my issues with chunks.

And dependability was key. I needed to blend poo daily and I wanted a blender that wouldn't pack it up in three goes. So to speak. Or in the middle of an infusion. Can you imagine? What would I ever do with a blender full of chunks of poo? I panicked at the thought of me racing around, looking for ways to get the mixture down the drain, chopping it up with a twig from the backyard or something. No, the blender could not break down. I would pay extra for a well-known, dependable brand. I stood in front of the blenders, quietly weighing their pros and cons, taking the time to figure out what I wanted, completely lost in my thoughts. This was for my son! He would get well!

"Can I help you?"

I jumped a mile.

"Just looking, thanks." Please god, make her go away. I still hadn't recovered from the officious sales help in the medical supply store.

"There are quite a few blenders on the market. Maybe I can help you digest all the information."

Digest? Did she really say that? And then what? Shit into a blender? Did she know?

Nah, impossible.

"Ah, no, that's okay, really. I'm just looking."

"What were you hoping to blend? Soups? Eggs? Sauces? Smoothies?"

I looked up at the ceiling trying to appear as though I was considering my answer. What I needed to blend wasn't on her list.

"Ah, good question," I said. I continued to ponder the ceiling.

She looked at me with that expectant, cheery look that idiots sometimes get.

"Smoothies," I finally said and then gained some momentum. "Mostly, chocolate smoothies." I was on a roll.

"I need to blend chunks of chocolate bars into smoothies."

Oh god, please let me die.

"Chunks? Hard chocolate chunks or soft? Chewy with peanuts? And will you be adding syrup as well?"

You know when you start to laugh and can't stop? This always happens to me when it shouldn't. At funerals. During speeches. Now.

It was the peanuts that set me off. I'd never be able to look at an Oh Henry! again.

My mouth emitted little squeaks. My body quivered. I turned my back and blew my nose. I took a breath. "All kinds of chunks. Hard ones, soft ones. Sometimes with syrup!"

The giggles bubbled into my throat and I turned my back, pretending to sneeze. It came out like a banshee wail as I roared with laughter.

She looked at me quizzically. "Do you need a spout on the blender to pour the smoothie into a glass?"

What? To drink? Jeezus. No!

But wait! I reconsidered. A spout might have its benefits. You never know. A spout could be helpful. I saw myself wearing an apron and daintily pouring the liquefied poo into an enema bag from a convenient spout.

"Is it easy to operate?"

"Yes, just pull this toggle towards you. No muss, no fuss."

"Ah. Sounds good. No muss is good." My fantasy might come true. But hold on. "Is the spout easy to clean?"

"Well, you have to undo the gizmo here and twist that nozzle there and pull the spout here…"

Meanwhile I'd be covered in shit.

"No thanks. The spout's a non-starter. I need something very easy and fast to clean."

This girl would not be daunted. She smiled, her lips curling to show her teeth. "The spouts are very good sellers, especially for people who use their blenders to make smoothies. It's so easy."

I shook my head. The spout was out. "No spout."

She asked smartly, "Any other criteria?"

"It needs to be made of glass."

She became all business again. "Oh, many of our customers prefer glass, it washes up so nice and clean and doesn't hold any residual odour, if you know what I mean."

"I can only imagine," I said. The giggles started up again. I gulped some air. Why was I so immature?

She rummaged through the shelves and finally threw me a box. Then she threw me a look.

"Here, I think this one is the one you need. Glass, easy to clean, plus it has enough wattage to do what sounds like quite a big job."

"Yes, it certainly is a big job. And I have one every morning."

Ha ha ha.

She ignored my shaking shoulders. I'm sure she had reached the conclusion, and rightly so, that the blender was for an asshole.

"You must think this blender is for an asshole." I was having so much fun.

She didn't reply and addressed me as if I were a naughty child, her finger pointing at the fine type on the packaging with her finger. "See here? I'm sure it will liquefy chunks." She underlined the next bit with her finger. "It says, 'Ten

speeds plus pulse function to handle every blending need.'"
She looked at me from under confident eyebrows as she
emphasized the word "every."

"*Every* blending need!" I mused thoughtfully. "Every
single one. Fancy that. Well, I'll be."

"You never know what you might need to blend one
day. What kind of chocolate bars do you use? Sweet
Marie? Coffee Crisp?"

I couldn't resist. "Tootsie Rolls." I looked at her
meaningfully. "Just today I read a recipe about making
a smoothie out of a Tootsie Roll. It called for peanuts.
Do you think this could handle that?"

"Oh sure, look at the name."

I read the name on the box and howled all the way to
the cash register. Bring on the poo! I would be undefeated.
Chunks would be destroyed! I was the proud owner of
a Black and Decker *Crush Master*.

7.
THE TRIAL RUN

THE FIRST TIME I made gravy I called my aunt and asked her how to do it. I said, "Hi Aunt Patty, how do you make gravy? I'm serving a roast chicken to my kids and gravy would be nice to go with it." She told me how: you know, drain the pan of excess fat, stir in flour, add water, whisk like crazy, add salt and bring to a boil. Her directions were clear and concise and I made great gravy, first time. I still make great gravy.

I couldn't really call my aunt about blending poo. I'm not putting her down or anything; I mean, my Aunt Patty can do everything — strip furniture, embroider, smock, put on a roof, make jam, wire her house. She's no slouch. But this? I'm not so sure she'd know how to do this. Imagine the conversation: "Hi Aunt Patty, my son hasn't been feeling that great lately ... remember he was diagnosed with Crohn's disease ... and remember when you told me how to make that great gravy? Well, I need to make a gravy again, only this time out of poo.... Yeah, you heard me, and then I want to shoot it up his bum. I need some pointers on collecting and whipping up the caca. Any ideas?"

I actually pondered for a day or two whether I should

make the call. I knew she'd be able to help me. She'd been a medic or something in Vietnam. And, as she said, I was always welcome to talk about crap with her. But I was just too chicken. I was too embarrassed. I couldn't ask her. No. I was on my own.

So I decided to do a trial run.

The day before the trial run I did a dry run. I put the toilet hat on the toilet rim, put the seat down, sat on the seat, and then put the female urinal in between my legs. I bent over and had a good look. Yeah, it looked like it would work. I was confident. Proud, in fact, of thinking of the female urinal. A stroke of genius. No pee in the poo for my son, no way!

I never thought this would be a goal of mine, right up there with losing thirty pounds. And stopping drinking.

To get ready for the infusion trial run, I ate a lot of vegetables at dinner and then a whole bowl of well-buttered popcorn. I drank about three beers. Okay, five. I was taking no chances. I was going to poo come hell or high water. The kids watched me stuff all this into my gob and told me I didn't have to stucco the side of the house.

The next morning the time was ripe and I dashed into the bathroom. I put the toilet hat on the rim. I put down the seat. I grabbed the female urinal. I sat down and spread my legs. I fit on the female urinal.

Holy crap! What a mess! First I washed my hands for far longer than the recommended ten seconds. Then I spent quite a long time cleaning up the bathroom floor, wiping down the side of the toilet and buffing the taps with antiseptic wipes. I finished by spraying my whole body with Lysol. Not really, but I felt like it. The toilet hat must have bitten me because there was a scrape on my bum. It was bleeding. How on earth did that happen?

So, that went well. Not.

I flung the stupid green vase/urinal and toilet hat into the recycling bin in the kitchen and frowned. It was all too complicated. I would just have to learn how to catch my poo in something else. What? A cookie tin? No, metal might contaminate the poo. A mason jar? What if it broke? Ouch. I mentally scrambled through my kitchen. Salad spinner? I tossed it aside. The egg boiling pot? The juice jug? And then I came to my big bin of disposable lunch containers. Ahhhh, I thought, now we're getting somewhere. Tupperware! I rummaged in the disposable container bin and came up with what I thought would be the perfect catcher. It was a square container about twice the depth of a sandwich container. It was the size I would use if I had to take a salad to work.

I needed to do another trial run. And fast. That day for lunch I ate a whole pound of fried mushrooms and garlic. We all have our Waterloo. By two in the afternoon I was in the toilet with Tupperware clamped to my bum.

I placed the plastic container perfectly with a corner in just the right location to miss getting pee in it. I was learning so much about anatomy. I slanted it just so. And then I looked at what I had done. It was perfect. I did it! There was only poo in the Tupperware. No pee! And as a bonus, there was no pee or poo on my hands.

I was ready to go, go go!

I took my new blender out of its box, washed the pieces and carefully dried them with a hair dryer. Perhaps I was being neurotic here, but Dr. Borody had said "no water" and I took him seriously. Also, I didn't want to use the tea towel to dry the bits. I knew the towel was clean, but *how* clean was a legitimate question in a house filled with animals and children. Then I assembled it. No, I didn't read the directions, I never read the instructions. Not even for my circular saw. That was a mistake and the wobbly table proved it.

I put on a pair of disposable gloves and muttered, "Hmmm, fits like a glove." I laughed at how witty I was.

And then I spooned the poo into the bottom of the blender.

Now for the sterile saline solution. I twisted off the little orange cap, thinking that was all I'd have to do. But no, underneath the cap the bottle was completely sealed. The solution inside the bottle had been completely sealed in. Sterile meant sterile! I spent some time trying to imagine how they did that at the factory and revelled in other major achievements of humanity such as getting the mint in peppermint patties. Somehow the liquid had got in, but how was I going to get it out? This was a test, I knew it. If I could get this bottle open then it would prove that I had an IQ that would qualify me for Mensa.

What would work? A knife? Nah, I'd end up stabbing myself. I took a beer bottle opener, a familiar tool that I just happened to have handy, and tried to flip the top part off. No go. So then I turned the opener around and used the pointy end one uses to puncture holes in tins of juice. I jabbed it in. The point dug into the plastic and made a small hole. I looked at the bottle opener. The point was encrusted with sticky apple juice. So much for "sterile."

I turned the bottle opener over, stuck the pointy end

in the small hole and levered it up. I was trying to make the hole bigger, but then suddenly the whole top of the bottle just snapped off! I yelped as the point punctured my skin. I shouted "NO!" as the opener flew out of my hands along with the bottle top and hit the far wall. I gasped as I grabbed the bottle just before it tilted onto its side.

Phew. All was safe.

I caught my breath and calmly poured the now open bottle of sterile saline solution over the poo until it was just covered. I am not an accurate cook with measurements at the best of times and I was guessing that this was enough.

Then I pressed "Liquefy." The blender roared into life and I watched with a sort of horrified glee as my poo turned into, well, frankly, it looked like gravy! I stared at it, thinking Aunt Patty would be proud of me for making such a smooth-looking gravy. Then I jolted back to reality.

The machine was roaring away, sounding like ten thousand dentist drills and it was time to stop the damn thing. I looked wildly for the off button. What, you can put ten buttons on a blender and one of them can't be called "Off?" I madly started punching all the buttons. I did this in various combinations. I was panicking. Three times "Crush Ice," one time "Whip." Four times "Blend," twice "Froth." The poo was churning up the sides. I needed to add more saline. I was breathing fast and hard now as my poo whirred around and around in the machine. Was I doomed to call in my neighbour, a smart guy who knew machines? What on earth would he think? Then I had a brainwave. I could unplug the damn thing. But then my finger randomly hit the "Pulse" button and the machine stopped as suddenly as it had started.

Peace descended upon the house. I filled my lungs with air. I opened a window. God, poo stunk.

I eased off the lid slowly, splattering only a bit onto the back wall, and, feeling like Betty Crocker, quaintly added more saline solution and a teaspoon of psyllium husks to the poo. I think I sang a cute tune like "whistle while you barf." Next I pushed "Liquefy" again until white caps frothed inside the blender. It was done. I supposed. How can one tell if whipped up poo is done? I took the blender off the machine part and removed the lid. It was ready to pour.

I tore open one of the transparent bags the disposable enema came in and lifted it slowly out. The long tube snaked away from me and I got a sense that severe difficulty was looming ahead. That snake would have to be tamed! I put the end of the tube into the sink and wedged the enema bag open. With one hand I held it open and with the other I poured in the slurry. I watched, fascinated, as it travelled down the tube and then miraculously stopped. Why did it do that?

My grade eleven physics class came rushing back to me. I could remember three things. Number one: nothing can be created or destroyed. Number two: I needed a smoke. And number three: For every action there is a reaction. As I lifted the bag up, poo slithered down the tube. As I lowered the bag, the poo retreated up the tube. It was like magic. I had a little fun playing teeter-totter with my bag of shit and then dumped everything into the sink.

Now for the clean up. I bunched the used bag up and folded it into a plastic shopping bag. The tube kind of spun around a bit before I could grab it and stuff it into the bag. I only got a few dribbles on the rug. The rug was one of those oatmeal coloured berber ones, so it didn't really show.

As I hunched over the sink washing the bits and pieces of the blender I nearly gagged. I needed air! The hot water was steaming away with clouds of odiferous fumes engulfing my face. I turned the tap off. Then I turned on the cold and washed everything in cold water. I knew this wasn't as sanitary as hot, but I had to live to tell the tale. What a stench! After everything was washed I rinsed it all in the hottest water I could stand and laid it prettily to dry on a towel folded by the sink, as if I'd been making brownies.

I pulled off my gloves, tossed them in the garbage bag, and tied it up tightly. With a magnificent gesture I threw the bag out. Ta dah! I had done it.

All I had to do was set the stage for putting the snake up my son's bum. No kid wants their mom to see their bum, so he needed a bed with a curtain around it. I let my mind ruminate on what I could use for a curtain as I opened up the futon in the basement and covered it with an old plastic tablecloth. Just in case. Then I put a sheet on top. I found some soft duvets and a pillow for his head. I needed to make a curtain with a split in it. I figured I could pass the snake in between the split to my son. Then he would have his privacy. I'd try not to look.

To make a curtain rod, I hammered one nail into the doorframe near the bed and another nail into the doorframe near the furnace room. I'd fix the holes later. When he was better. He was going to get better, wasn't he? I hoped and hoped that he would be well as I worked.

SKY CURTIS

Then I found a piece of rope and threaded it through the hem of two old sheets. I tied one end of the rope up, then the other. The curtain fell just in front of the bed. I felt so smart. He had his very own privacy screen. I was completely ready.

My dress rehearsal had been successful. There would be no surprises.

And just what would the Chief of Medicine think of me now?

78

8.

THE FIRST INFUSION

EVERYTHING WAS READY for the first infusion, except we still didn't know if I could be a donor. I lifted the phone and nervously dialed the alternate doctor's office. It was the day before Christmas and if I didn't get an answer on my blood and poo results today, Chris would have to wait about ten more days before we could commence the infusions. And he was failing more every day. Anyone who has watched someone in the middle of a flare up knows that you can actually see the weight fall away, a bit every day. He was down about thirty pounds. I hoped against hope the test results were in.

After a runaround with the doctor's answering machine, the secretary finally called me back at about ten to five.

"Mrs. Curtis? Your blood results came back and they're fine. You are good to go."

I held the phone away from my face while I laughed. Did she actually say I was good to *go*?

"Thanks. But what about the liver tests?"

For the past week I'd had visions of the lab technician trying to catch the vial of blood for the liver test. I saw her racing around the lab with a net in her hand. We won't even go into how much alcohol I'd consumed over the course of my life. More than enough. Way, way more than enough.

"Your liver is fine."

"It's a miracle." I vowed, right then and there, that I would stop drinking. I had dodged a major bullet.

She faxed the set of results and I scanned them carefully. My B12 was good. No hepatitis. No AIDS. Iron, good. But what was that? I peered closer at the list. A checkmark against the Epstein Barr virus? I was positive for Epstein Barr? That wasn't good. I couldn't give my son Epstein Barr. He already slept forty hours a day! The infusion was off! Why was I told I could go ahead? But I didn't feel tired.

I called my regular family doctor in a panic. With luck she'd still be in. She explained I could have had Epstein Barr at any time, even years ago, perhaps while I was a young child. She said that even though I had the antigens, that didn't mean I had the virus now. I felt a huge relief. This meant that we could go ahead. Tomorrow. December 25th.

Merry Christmas.

Many kids wake up Christmas morning and charge around the tree, flinging wrappings hither and yon. Many moms are in the kitchen, basting the turkey and shoving stuffing up its bum. Me? Well, something would be going up a bum, and it wasn't stuffing, although my son was a bit of a turkey. There he was, lying on the futon, hiding behind the curtains I'd rigged up. Gloves, K-Y Jelly and Kleenex were close at hand.

I was in the basement bathroom, doing my thing with a Tupperware container.

This was not, by any stretch of the imagination, your typical Christmas morning. But if it worked? What a gift!

Job done, I put on a pair of gloves and spooned it into a blender. We all know what "it" is. I covered it with sterile saline solution, added a teaspoon of psyllium husks and pressed "Liquefy."

I'd like everyone to know that it's really important to put the lid of the blender on tightly. I rapidly pressed "Pulse" and the roaring stopped. There were just a few splashes on the wall, but hey, no biggie, I'd clean that up later. Christmas gravy goes everywhere too. In the distance I heard "Jingle Bells" and some thumping. I guessed the girls were jumping around upstairs, all excited because it was Christmas morning. I poured in more sterile solution, gave the blender a shake, put the lid on very tightly this time because I learn quickly and pressed "Liquefy" again.

Once the solution was frothy, I put the end of the tube attached to the enema bag into the sink, held the bag down lower than the end of the tube (I'd learned my physics lesson!) and poured my Christmas gift to my son into the bag.

This year he was getting a bag of shit.

I closed the top of the bag with the handy zip-lock fastener and grabbed the end of the tube. As I walked toward him, I briefly forgot about keeping the end of the tube higher than the bag, but I wouldn't forget again.

How *does* one get poo out of carpet anyway?

I parted my ingenious curtains slightly and stuck the snake end in between the crack saying, "Ready?"

Chris grunted.

"Gloves on? K-Y at hand?"

He grunted again. I didn't think he was enjoying this much. I heard blankets rustling.

I stood outside the curtain in some bizarre yoga pose, one hand holding a bag of poo close to the ground and the other waving the end of a brown-filled tube over my head. I could feel poo dripping down my arm. Great. My back was beginning to ache. My upper hand was going a bit numb as the blood rushed into my head. I could hear it pounding in my ears.

"Ready?" I asked shrilly.

Nothing. He still hadn't taken the tube. I waited. I heard rustling. More rustling. Even more rustling. What was he doing? Then he took the tube from me and I waited long enough to be sure it was in him. The rustling finally stopped. It must be in him. I stood up straight, feeling my back creak.

Chris shouted, "Lower the bag, lower the bag, lower the stupid bag!"

Gobs of poo ran down the curtain. I heard the Kleenex box being rapidly emptied. The basement stunk worse than a barn. It seemed I had made an assumption that the end of the tube was in where it was supposed to be.

It wasn't.

"Sorry, honey."

Upstairs a tape played. "Rudolph the Red Nosed Reindeer."

I was gripped with laughter but knew I couldn't let it out. My poor boy. I'm sure my humour was a coping mechanism for knowing how terribly ill he was. I was coping very well, laughing my head off, but trying not to.

More rustling. Then, "Okay, you can lower the bag."

I watched the level of the slurry go down in the bag as it went into my son.

I am sure there are moments in everyone's lives where there is a pause and a reflection of one's actions. I had one of those moments right then. I could see the cameras rolling, taking a movie of a crazy lady holding a bag of poo up high, watching it as it emptied into her son.

What on earth was I doing?

But I trusted Dr. Borody. Human probiotic infusions made so much sense. But it was so bizarre. If you thought about it. I tried not to think about it.

And then the level in the bag stopped going down. Was he full up? "Are you full of shit, honey?"

"Ha ha. It's stopped coming out."

"What do you mean?"

"I mean, it's stopped coming out."

"It's stopped coming out?

"That's what I said."

"Oh."

Now what? An airlock?

I squeezed the bag. It wouldn't squeeze.

"I think it's stuck." I panted as I pumped the bag up and down, trying to get the stuff to come out.

"Stuck? What with?

"Maybe an airlock."

"Did you blend it long enough? I think maybe there are chunks."

Chunks!

Of course! I knew it!

"Take it out and I'll go reblend it."

"Reblend isn't a word."

"It is now," I shouted through the curtain. I was furious. I had paid extra for the Crush Master blender. There should be no chunks. My poor son had to stick the tube in him *again*. Already his bum was sore and bleeding. I silently said 'Damn damn damn" as I went back to my infusion station, carrying my slimy enema bag.

I reblended the slurry and we started over. It went well for about three minutes. Then the slurry got stuck again. Meanwhile, my glasses seemed to be smeared. Good thing I'd worn them, that's all I could think.

"You probably have enough in you; let's call it a day. Hold it in."

"Hold it in?"

"Ya, Dr. Borody said for at least an hour."

"An hour?" he shouted as he raced to the toilet.

Hmm, I thought. That went well.

9.

THE FIRST FEW WEEKS

WITH A FEW DAYS of practice the infusion process became streamlined. Not perfect, not by a long shot, but over the course of the first week we managed to get some of the slurry into my son. I worried because he couldn't manage to keep the slurry in for very long. Twenty minutes seemed to be the maximum time. Was this long enough? I had no idea. After seven daily infusions we started doing them once a week, as we had been instructed by Dr. Borody.

I lived in a state of constant fear during this time. Chris wasn't doing well at all. He had a high fever and woke up every night, several times, covered in sweat. I had a pile of clean sheets and duvets beside his bed so our nocturnal bed makings were easier. The laundry was never ending and I would put the linen in the washing machine, trying not to see the bloodstains.

I was on the phone daily to Dr. Borody in Australia, his soothing voice and rounded vowels calming me down. God knows what time it was in Australia. Probably four in the morning. I was so grateful that this man was a dedicated doctor, only wanting to help someone who was very ill. I was so worried about Chris's fever.

"What if my poo has given him a horrible disease? He's gone septic? My bacteria has leached through his intestinal wall? He has ulcers in his intestines. They're open and bleeding. I am very frightened."

Dr. Borody was reassuring. "His own poo doesn't hurt him. Neither does yours. Having a fever is normal. How high is it? "

"I don't know, we don't have a thermometer, but I think it might be about 103."

"It will go down. How does he feel?"

"He seems to be okay, actually, just hot."

"Is he up and walking around? Or can't he get his head off the pillow?"

"Oh no, he's up. He's walking around. Watching a movie."

"It will go down."

Two days later it did. I was so relieved. He still woke up in sweats and I tried to tell myself it was the disease leaving his body. Was it?

But the next serious problem we had to deal with was gas. And not just a little. Chris's stomach was bloated as if he were six months pregnant. He was tooting every two minutes. I say tooting because that's the polite way to describe what sounded like a train thundering through the house. I wondered why Chris didn't fly around the room like a deflating balloon. We won't even go into the smell. I looked in the yellow pages for gas masks. When I told someone this they thought I was kidding.

I was on the phone again. "Dr. Borody, he has terrible, terrible gas. Room clearing farts. It's unbelievable. He could be used in chemical warfare and destroy entire armies."

"His bacteria is getting reorganized. This is normal. If it's really bad, take out the psyllium husks. The bacteria are feeding on them and making gas."

Ah ha! I knew the psyillium husks were just supplementary!

We took the husks out of the slurry recipe and the gas sort of disappeared. Chris's stomach shrank to the size of about a three-month pregnant belly and the smell settled down to about five dozen rotten eggs.

And then the next problem surfaced. My son was lying in bed covered in sweat and looking at me beseechingly. The sheets were drenched. The mattress was sodden. His skin was flushed. He was moaning that he was on fire. I touched his cheek. Cool as a cucumber. I called Dr. Borody. Again.

"This is why we use male donors. My donors for human probiotic infusions are always male. Female poo has female hormones in it. Think about it. Women go through a lot because of their hormones. Their breasts balloon. I had one patient whose wife was a donor while she was pregnant. He was sick as a dog. Threw up every morning. And when women are going through menopause? They don't sleep, they gain weight, they pee a lot, they get really, really crabby. And they have hot flashes. How old are you?"

"I've been through menopause." I felt like Joan Rivers keeping my age a secret. No way I was going to tell him how old I was!

"And now so has he. It will go away, over time, as his body adjusts. And then it will adjust back."

Most kids who get Crohn's are in their early twenties,

right? This would make their mothers about, oh, that charming menopausal age of fifty to fifty-five. And if you're trying to cure a male with the poo from a menopausal woman? Well, well, well, how interesting. Poor Chris. I guess when he gets married he'll have a certain sympathy for his wife when she's going through menopause. He'll know exactly what she means when she says, "I'm having hot flashes."

If he was ever well enough to get married. Or do any of those things one does before that time, like go to school, have a girlfriend, get a job. Hell, I'd be happy if he could walk!

The infusions were certainly having an effect on my very ill son, but my heart constricted when I faced the reality that they weren't really working. Although I was always hopeful, I knew there was the reality of what was going on with his body. Chris was still pooing blood twenty times a day. This was nowhere near normal. But then, it was better than it had been, somewhat of an improvement, down from forty. Plus, he wasn't gaining weight. He was a bag of bones. I kept the mirrors hidden and the scale in a closet. But then, on the other hand, he had stopped losing weight. It was holding steady. He still had painful mouth cankers, but the boils on his legs were going away. There were no new ones. Plus his joint pain was gone. The fever was mostly non-existent, although every now and then it flared up.

But the truth of the matter was the infusions hadn't really worked. He wasn't *better*. Not even close.

I was beside myself. They *had* to work. He had to get completely better. I got in my car and drove around and around the city, up one block, down another, on the highway, back again, mulling it over and over. They *had* to work. There was absolutely no reason why they shouldn't. Besides, they were working a little. There were a few good signs. But I had to face the truth. He was still a very sick boy.

If Crohn's was caused by a bacterial infection, then infusions would cure it. There was almost a hundred percent cure rate for C. difficile using infusions. Why not MAP? Or whatever bacteria caused these huge ulcers in my poor son's intestines.

I *knew* Crohn's disease was caused by an infection. I just didn't believe in that autoimmune disease stuff. Call me twisted and bitter, but I believed that concept was made up by doctors who couldn't take responsibility for destroying a person's internal flora with antibiotics. Or had no other explanation for a disease.

I knew it because when Chris had been on the anti-MAP antibiotic therapy for a year, he had been completely better. In my mind, the ulcers were caused by bacteria. On the skin. Under the skin. In the intestine.

My mind went in circles as I drove in circles. Over and over I reviewed the little I knew. Duodenal ulcers were caused by bacteria. That had been proven. Plus, if antibiotics for MAP worked, which they did, then Crohn's was also caused by a bacteria. Had to be. Infusions worked for C. difficile. Infusions *had* to work for Crohn's or whatever disease Chris had. The theory of good bacteria crowding out and killing off bad bacteria had to apply to all bacteria in general. Infusions made so much sense.

As I drove around the city I came to the conclusion we

were doing it wrong. Dr. Borody's protocol wasn't quite right for Crohn's/colitis. It worked for constipation, IBS, other causes of diarrhea, but Crohn's/colitis? Not so much.

I had never felt so alone in my life. What was I going to do now? I had to get my son better. The infusions simply had to work. Why didn't the Canadian medical system have any help for this? When I got home I Googled doctors who were doing infusions for C. difficile. There weren't that many of them and I wrote down the phone number of a guy who worked in Oshawa, close to Toronto.

The next morning I called and carefully explained the situation to the medical receptionist and then asked if I could bring my son in to see the doctor. She called me back saying that the doctor said I should go back to the gastro, he only dealt with infectious diseases.

I hissed into the phone, "Crohn's IS an infectious disease." And slammed it down. Goddam fucking doctors. So stupid. Of course it was an infectious disease! That's why it responds to antibiotics. Geezus.

So, I was on my own. Now what?

10.

FIGURING IT OUT

I KNEW we were doing something wrong and I needed to figure out how to do it right. I would not give up. I would NOT.

It made too much sense. Dr. Borody's protocol was a good start. There were some improvements in Chris's health, his swollen ankle had gone down, his knee had stopped hurting, there were no new boils or cankers, but pooing blood twenty times a day was not *better*. The improvements weren't enough to say that the infusions had worked. Not even close. My mind whirred over all the various things we could try to get the damn things to really work. There were so many 'maybes.'

Maybe we weren't doing it enough. Maybe Chris was so ill he needed three times as many infusions. Maybe he needed to stand on his head while he did them. And I wasn't kidding when I thought about this. Maybe that would help the slurry cover more of his intestine and heal it. Maybe he needed to eat only brown rice. Maybe this, maybe that.

I wasn't going to give up. No way. I believed in the infusions. I believed the disease was called by bacteria. I didn't believe in autoimmune diseases. I had utter faith in the human body's innate drive to be well. I did not believe that the body would attack itself for no reason. If it were attacking itself, it was trying to fight off an infection. That was my theory and I was sticking to it. But what did I know? I didn't have years of medical school under my belt. I was just a mother!

I sat at my computer and Googled everything I could think of. Fecal this. Transplant that. Bacteria. MAP. Human Probiotic Infusions. Crohn's. Colitis. Everything under the sun that had to do with intestinal diseases. It took me hours and hours. I was on a quest for an answer: why weren't the infusions working and what did I have to do to get them to work?

Finally, a few days later, I came across a tiny tidbit of information buried deep in an article that made some sense to me. I read that there was some speculation that it was hard for new bacteria to colonize in an intestine filled with ulcers. It needed healthy lining to latch onto. I remembered Chris's colonoscopy pictures and knew that if this were true, then nothing would be able to find a home in those gaping wounds. Chris's intestine was filled with ulcers.

This information got me thinking. It was all about the bacteria recolonizing. So, it was my job to make a nice home for the new bacteria so it could get settled. Keeping the home stable so the new baby bacteria could move right in and thrive. I was a mother, I understood at least this.

So, I started to think about the healthy bacteria trying to colonize. Well, clearly the state of the intestines was pretty key and would have to be addressed, but what about the constant pooing? How on earth could new healthy bacteria have even a chance of colonizing if it didn't stay in the intestine for longer than five minutes? How could new bacteria colonize if it was constantly being pooed out? This was like asking someone into your home for a cup of tea and shooing them out the door before the kettle even boiled. And the state of Chris's intestines? It was as if we were asking someone into a home for a nice visit without giving them any furniture to sit on in a room full of toxic waste. And then rushing them out the door before they even said boo!

Of course this was why the infusions weren't working. Why didn't I think of all this before? All that pooing. All that bleeding. All that raw intestine with no lining. It made so much sense to me. So, how to solve the problem? How to create a nice home for the new bacteria? One where there was at least something to sit on and where they could hang around for an hour or so, get settled and make themselves at home.

I might not be a doctor, but I knew how to entertain my guests! Give them a glass of wine. Help them relax. Create a quiet atmosphere that was conducive for meaningful conversation. Put on some nice music, feed them a delicious meal. Smooth out the rough edges of everyone's day. Let them stay as long as they want. Laugh, feel no pain! Have a nice time.

Simply put, we needed DRUGS!

Chris needed drugs while doing the infusions. He needed drugs to help heal the ulcers. To stop the pooing. To help him rest. To keep him out of pain. To smooth the rough edges. To get rid of those raw deep cankers and split anal fissures. I talked to him about my theory. He lay and bed and looked like he had given up hope. With every one of his sighs, I chattered even more excitedly, trying to cheer him up, trying to make him see the logic.

"I think this will work sweetie. We have to be nice to our guests. The bacteria is like company and we have to make it feel at home. Furniture. Food. Encourage them to hang around. Get it?"

Chris turned his head towards the wall. "Whatever."

"No, I mean it. Get rid of the inflammation. Bring on the steroids. Stop the diarrhea. Surely there's a drug for that. Get rid of the mouth ulcers. Something has to do that. Heal the anal fissures. Surely there's a cream. End the cycle of pain. Take a great painkiller. Help you sleep. Use sleeping pills. We're going to get you better, honey, and I'm sure this will work."

"If you say so."

"I do say so. You just watch me."

We immediately upped Chris's Prednisone to 40 mg a day. No, I didn't ask the doctor if this was a good thing to do. I knew it was. Doctors are so weird about Prednisone. Even the mention of it and they start tut-tutting as if it were poison. It's a great little drug. It works. It gets rid of inflammation like a treat. So he started taking eight of the little white bombs. He wasn't happy about this because they made him so jittery, but the ulcers had to go. He took them in the morning so he could sleep at night. Luckily Chris didn't have the moonfaced reaction to Prednisone that most people get. Besides, we knew he'd come off them eventually.

Because this would work.

After five years of having Crohn's, he knew his body very well. He had a sense of what was going on in it. He said he needed a steroid enema. As he put it, he needed something on site. I didn't question his judgment. Off I trotted to my friendly pharmacist and talked to her about various products. She ran her finger down a page in a book until she found what she was looking for. She told me she thought Entocort was a good steroid enema on the market. I dutifully wrote it down. I asked her if it could be taken in conjunction with Prednisone. She read the fine print and said yes.

I talked to her about a mouth rinse that cancer patients use when chemotherapy causes mouth cankers, Apo-Benzydamine. My friend's mother unfortunately had to use it and had had great success with the drug. The pharmacist checked her stock and waved a bottle of green liquid victoriously in front of me. She had some!

I asked her how people usually stop diarrhea and she walked from behind the counter to the shelves stocked with packages of over the counter drugs. She tapped a package of Imodium with her fingernail. Imodium? It seemed so obvious, so run of the mill. Shouldn't we use a fancy anti-runs drug? But no, the best thing was an over the counter, ages old product, Imodium. I grabbed three packages. She raised her eyebrows. I shrugged.

I discussed his pain level. It was very bad. He was writhing on the bathroom floor or lying down in the shower with nice warm water pulsing on his belly. He was in a great deal of pain. Every now and then he was reduced to tears. My heart wept as I stood by helplessly, watching him huddle his body into itself. I hated the pain. He said he hated his life. I needed this disease to go away so badly. We had to control the pain.

The pharmacist agreed with me that a serious antacid would lessen his pain symptoms. She said that Losec, a drug that prevented acid secretion, would help. I asked her if people ever took twice the recommended amount. She nodded and said yes.

We had quite a long conversation about painkillers. Morphine? Medical marijuana? She said to start with plain old regular Tylenol and see how that worked. She told me to give him two every four hours, around the clock, whether or not he was in pain because pain was a cycle and it had to be broken. She told me to stay ahead of the pain and that when I was completely sure it was lessening, to drop down to one every four hours. I bought a large bottle.

I talked to her about his anal fissures. I told her they were so painful that my son said they felt like paper cuts, only you know where. She said he probably needed the brand of Anusol that had a steroid in it. I wrote that down. I was making a list to take to the alternative doctor who had told us about Dr. Borody and his treatments.

I talked to her about his nausea level. He could hardly eat because everything made him feel like throwing up. She said the 24-hour Gravol worked well and would help calm his stomach down. It too was an over-the-counter drug.

I left the drug store armed with Tylenol, Gravol and Imodium. As soon as I got home I faxed our supportive alternative doctor, for prescriptions for more Prednisone, Losec, Anusol with steroids, Entocort and the

Apo-Benzydamine. She was so kind, so supportive, so outside the realm of a normal Canadian doctor that I knew she would fax the prescriptions to the pharmacist. It would take a few hours for the prescriptions to be filled, so while I waited I started Chris on the new over-the-counter drugs.

I read the cautions on the box of Imodium with dismay. They said not to use the product when blood and mucus were present in the diarrhea. I shrugged and said pshaw. We would risk it. It said not to take more than six a day. I uttered another pshaw. We would risk that too. He always had diarrhea right after he ate and he ate four times a day. So Chris took two about twenty minutes before each meal and then two at night before his snack. If he woke up, he'd take two more. When we saw how well it worked, I bought it in bulk at Walmart. It worked perfectly, calming down his constant urge to go from every hour to about four times a day. The new bacteria would now have half a chance to recolonize.

We began dosing him up with the Tylenol and the relief was immediate. Every four hours without fail all day long he took two regular Tylenol. Every morning with the Prednisone I gave him a long-lasting Gravol. He went back to sleep. Finally Chris was resting.

That afternoon I picked up the filled prescriptions and Chris started on all those medications as well. He looked skeptically at the green gargle and I knew I was going to run into a problem here. Chris had this thing about drugs killing him. No wonder. He'd had an anaphylactic reaction to the liquid Benadryl in his Remicade that had frightened him unbelievably. So I told him about our friend's mother taking it and how well it had worked for her. He just looked at me. I told him to put just a little on his tongue first, to try it out. He wouldn't. So I put some on a tablespoon and swished it around in my mouth to prove that it wouldn't kill him. I didn't tell him it tasted like hand sanitizer.

My strategy worked. Finally he grabbed the bottle by the neck and knocked some back into his mouth. He swished it around so it touched the inside of his cheeks. He did this again later that night and the cankers that had plagued him for months simply disappeared. They were gone the next morning! It was magic. I was flabbergasted. What was in that stuff? The fine print was covered up by the prescription label. Would it work on his intestinal ulcers as well? I emailed Dr. Borody and asked if Chris could swallow the stuff.

He emailed me back quickly: No! Poison!

Silly me.

Then I read the package for the steroid Anusol. It said to use after every bowel movement. You gotta be kidding. Opening up the foil wrapping would become a full time occupation. The twelve little suppositories would last less than a day. So, Chris put them in a few times a day and then before bed.

Chris was prescribed a six-week supply of Entocort, the steroid enema, and that night he squirted one in. He held it in as long as he could, knowing the steroids would heal up the inflammation. After he squirted it out, he put in a steroid Anusol suppository. Chris became the steroid king! He rattled with drugs.

I climbed the stairs to his bedroom that night to make

sure Chris had settled in for the night. He hadn't had a full night's sleep in months, pooing blood every hour or two. The Imodium had helped with this, but he desperately needed a good night's sleep to heal. I believed in the power of sleep to heal the body and regretted not asking the doctor for some sleeping pills. And then I remembered that I had a little stash in my bedside table. I had hidden behind my reading glasses a very small bottle of ten little Ativan pills, a highly addictive anti-anxiety medication that had been prescribed to me for emergencies.

This was one of those emergencies. I went back down the stairs, snatched the bottle, and carefully doled out one to Chris. That night he slept like a baby, between the Imodium and the Ativan. I didn't hear him coming down the stairs once. Now we were getting somewhere.

Shakespeare's line, "Sleep knit up the ravelled sleeve of care" crossed my mind the next morning when Chris came downstairs, looking rested for the first time in months. Sleeping is such a healing thing to do.

But he said his stomach "kinda" hurt, and I guessed it was probably because of all the medication. I gave him not one but two Losec to take with the Prednisone. I watched him throw a handful of pills into his mouth. Would this strategy work? Just one day had gone by and he said he was already feeling a bit better. I could tell he was relaxing a bit as the pain level subsided.

Now we had to get the infusion method a little more user friendly. It had to become far easier to do. The enema bag system was not a good one for an adolescent boy and his mother! And clearly, seven infusions once a day in a row and then once a week for a month was not an infusion protocol that would work on Chris's Crohn's disease. That was the next step that would have to be figured out.

11.

NEW INFUSION PROTOCOL

THE INFUSIONS had *sort of* worked but the schedule for infusions didn't seem long enough. I needed better than "*sort of* worked." I figured we weren't doing it enough. The protocol of seven infusions and then one a week for a month wasn't going to do the job on poor, very sick Chris. He had it BAD. I knew that one shot of slurry for C. difficile often worked, but this MAP was stubborn. Apparently this bacteria is one in a handful of bacteria that reproduces by spores instead of by splitting. These spores are encased in a shell so hard that not even fire can break it down. That's why this particular bacteria is very difficult to get rid of. The only thing that could kill off the spores are antigens in human stool. That was my understanding, anyway.

It also struck me that seven days of any treatment was often not enough to turn any infection around. Even the antibiotics I was familiar with from my children being sick when they were little were often prescribed for two weeks. Plus, there was always that warning on the bottle to take all the medication until finished. This was to make sure that all the bacteria had been killed off.

With this sophisticated scientific background, ha ha, I

decided that we needed to do way more infusions than just once a day for seven days. We had to keep doing the infusions until the bad bacteria was all gone.

I talked to Chris and asked him if he minded doing an infusion every day for a month. "This is a very serious disease. It needs a very serious attack!"

"Okay."

Hmmm, I thought. That was easy. But then again, it wasn't as if he was going anywhere, being confined to bed. "And I think we have to give the disease a great deal of respect. It has the ability to hang around a long time. Its spores are made of steel!"

"Okay."

He was on his computer. Probably Facebook.

"I think we need to do it daily for a month and then every second day for three weeks then every third day for three weeks and then every fourth day for three weeks and so on, until we get to one a week for three weeks, then one every two weeks for three weeks, and then one a month for three months. At least."

"Okay." He typed away.

"Look at me. Put that computer down."

"Can't Mom, I'm designing websites. If I can't go out and work, I'll work from my bed."

My heart just swelled with pride. Such a resilient kid! "Where'd you learn to do that? You're designing websites? I'm so proud of you honey, but did you hear a word I said? I would like it if we could get you out of bed. We are talking about a major commitment to infusions here if we're going to get rid of this infection."

Chris looked down at his emaciated body and then at

me. He sighed. "Sure, Mom. I'm game for it."

We both knew this was his last chance at getting better or else lose his intestine and poo into a bag for the rest of his life. Or else be sick three months out of six. Or else never have a normal life. Or else not eat regular food ever again. Every avenue that the medical profession had provided to us has been exhausted. "That's great honey. It may be over kill, so to speak, but better that than under kill. "

"Okay, Mom. I'm kinda busy here." He reached for his computer.

He was always in a rush, that boy. I said, "Just a minute more. I have to talk to you about the enema bag."

"Yeah, well, that has to go. It's messy. It's embarrassing. It's unreliable. The little hole hurts my intestines, the edges of it scrapes as the tube goes in and scrapes on the way out."

When he told me this I cringed. Why hadn't he said something earlier? The enema bag hurt him? That was stupid. It had to go. "Okay honey, no more enema bag and the plastic snake. I'll think of something."

I left his room, hearing the tapping of keys behind me. I pondered the question of the day: how does one squirt slurry up a bum? I needed a new kind of gizmo. What were the options?

A turkey baster?

An oiling can?

I had no idea what was available to me. What was available on the market for this task alone was hardly a question I could ask the sales person in the medical supply store.

I fantasized my shopping experience. "Excuse me miss, would you like to shoot the shit? Yes? And just how would you like to do that?"

I definitely was not going to ask that question. No matter how helpful, how professional they were at the medical supply store, I would have to solve this problem on my own. I had to browse up and down the aisles and physically touch stuff, examine it slowly. Off I went to the medical supply store, hoping to avoid Attila the Sales Person.

And if I couldn't find something that worked there, I'd try out the hardware store. I would find something that worked better than an enema bag.

I meandered up and down the aisles, finally standing in front of the needle section. Talk about selection. Large ones, small ones, curved ones. I rejected those immediately. I contemplated the base of needles, giving their plungers a hopeful squeeze. That would work, I thought, but way too small an amount. Even the biggest one wouldn't hold enough slurry. I figured at least 100 cc had to go in. Or four or five ounces. But maybe Chris could do it a few times to get enough in. I ran my thumb around the edge of the base to see if it would hurt going in. My thumb felt the hard corner of the edge, no wouldn't work. Way too sharp.

"Looking for something specific?" asked a cute little sales clerk.

"No," I waved my hand airily, "Just browsing."

I hoped I had said this the way one does when one is trying to be polite, but really wants the sales help to vanish into a cloud of smoke.

"If you need help, just find me." She wandered off.

"Thanks," I said gratefully to her retreating back.

I went back to exploring the needles. No, they simply wouldn't work.

Next I stood in front of the syringe aisle. They were the human version of a turkey baster. You could buy a female kind that had a rounded end with lots of little tiny holes. The construction was right, but no way would the infusion get through those miniscule holes. Plus the bag thing was too big. I wanted something that Chris could do on his own.

Right next to the female syringes were rectal syringes. Hmm. Sounded good.

I gravitated toward them like a thirsty traveler to an oasis on a desert. Had I found Mecca? I opened up the box and lifted one out. I squeezed the bulb, half expecting it to honk. It was big enough to hold a decent squirt. Then I examined the little nozzle and held the hole right up to my eye. Would the infusion go through that? Probably not. Chunks. I turned it over in my hand, thinking. It was tapered. I could cut it off half way up the tube where it was wider and get a larger hole.

Would it cut with a regular serrated knife? I could see myself sawing away, holding it down on a cutting board. I would smooth out the jagged end by heating the tube end on the stove and pressing the sharp bits in with my thumb. But what if something went wrong? What if I set the house on fire? Try explaining *that* to the fire department.

Or what if the tube cracked as I sawed away? So I put two in my basket. Then I thought about it and tossed in a third. Better to be safe than sorry.

I went home and hacked at the nozzle. I heated up the jagged end on the stove burner and smoothed it down. I pushed my new nozzle back into the tube and handed it to Chris with bated breath.

"You got to be kidding."

"What, you don't think it will work?"

"It'll work okay, but I won't put that up my bum. It will kill."

"But I smoothed out the edges."

"No."

"You could use K-Y Jelly on it."

"No."

He had that look which meant there was no way I would be able to convince him to use this jerry rigged rectal syringe. I took a new one out of the box and handed it to him. "What about this?"

"Ya, I could use that."

So, now the problem became getting the infusion mixture thin enough to go through what was quite a small hole. Now, finally it was time to deal with the dreaded fact.

Chunks.

It was time for me to face this major issue. It was a problem and I had to stop living in denial. The Crush Master could only do so much.

I called Dr. Borody.

"I seem to be having a problem with chunks getting stuck in the tubing." It was a small lie as we had ditched the tubing, but I was talking very long distance and I didn't want to go into the whole forgetting the enema bag bit and trying a new rectal syringe. The answer would be the same. I knew it would help.

"Oh yeah," he replied in his rounded Australian accent. "My nurse sometimes puts the tube on the floor and rolls a broom over it.

How hi tech I thought.

"A broom."

"Yes, she rolls it over the tube and flattens out the chunks until they can go through."

"Flattens them out."

He must have sensed my unwillingness to try this method. He snapped, "Some people strain the infusion mixture."

Now we were getting somewhere. "Strain it?"

He was impatient. Perhaps I sounded like an idiot parrot. "One of those mesh strainers." He said it as if I lived in the backwoods and had never seen one.

"Yes, we have them here. I keep one in my tent."

He laughed. "Try that."

"But the mixture would be so thin."

"Doesn't matter. Some people use coffee filters."

My mind boggled with the hundreds of replies I could make to that, like, 'My, your coffee tastes like shit.'

But I said nothing. I had my solution. A strainer. I'd buy a new one. Of course I would.

"Chris seems to have trouble keeping the enema in."

"Tell him to keep his hips up."

"His hips up?"

"Yes, on a pillow. He can put his legs up the wall. Then there's no pressure on his rectum and it will stay in."

Such a simple solution to a problem that had plagued Chris ever since the start of the infusions. When I told Chris he rolled his eyes. "Why didn't he tell us that at the very beginning?"

"He thought we knew."

"How would I know *that*?"

I reread the home infusion instructions he had sent, and there it was, in black and white: elevate the hips. I felt terrible that I had missed this very key piece of information. But then I cut myself some slack. My mind had been so very preoccupied. I was living in a state of fear. And grief.

Just what would my conservative husband say about all this?

The next morning I took the nozzle off a new unadulterated syringe and washed the rubber ball out with hot soapy water, getting it nice and clean on the inside for use. It seemed a bit ironic, all that effort to get it clean and then filling it with poo. I'd been to school. I knew the definition of irony I thought as I shook soapy water around and around to finally squirt it out and rinse, rinse, rinse.

But then I realized that I couldn't dry out the inside of the bulb. What to do? I squeezed the bulb of the syringe as tightly as I could, folding it into itself. When I let go I could hear air sucking into the bulb. I'd be at it for hours, if this was how I was going to air dry the inside of the bulb. But, it followed if I squeezed it tightly and then stuck the open end of the bulb into the sterile solution, it would suck it up. The inside of the syringe might be wet, but with something that wouldn't harm the bacteria. I opened the bottle of sterile solution, put some in a bowl, squeezed the syringe and sucked some up. I swirled it around and then squirted it out. There.

I whipped up some poo and sterile solution in the blender and poured it through my new strainer into a plastic container. I swirled it around, inspecting for chunks. Couldn't see any, but then, you know how they are.

Now it was time to fill 'er up! I squeezed the bulb as tightly as I could and put the open end of the syringe into the infusion. I let go of my hand and watched with great satisfaction as it sucked the infusion up with a small sigh. The syringe was filled almost completely. Things were looking good.

Then I stuck on the nozzle by twisting it into the hole. I quickly learned that while one is putting the nozzle into the bulb, it is very, very important to not squeeze the bulb. Rather, one should gently rest the bulb in one hand while maneuvering the nozzle into the hole with the other. I repeated to myself, do not squeeze the bulb. It took me ten minutes to change my shirt and start over. I had saved my Tupperware of slurry just in case something like this happened.

Once the nozzle was in the bulb I gave it a tentative squeeze. The infusion blasted out in a thin propelled stream like there was no tomorrow. It worked! I cleaned off the counter top with some paper towel and Lysol and rinsed the bulb off carefully, making sure I didn't get any water into the nozzle. Then I put the bulb into a mug with the nozzle facing up and carried it up the stairs to my son. It just happened to be a mug with a Campbell's soup logo on it.

"Here honey, here's your cup of poop."

He looked at me as if I'd lost my mind.

"Squeeze this in, just like you were putting in one of your steroid enemas."

He looked dubiously at the bulb and nozzle.

"It'll work," I reassured him. "Cover the nozzle with K-Y."

He raised an eyebrow at me. I don't think he liked me discussing his private parts so intimately.

I rambled on. "Then, once it's in, put your hips on a pillow and your feet up the wall. It will stay in. Keep it in for as long as you can."

"I'll need Kleenex, gloves, and a garbage pail." he said, acting like he was a king demanding peeled grapes. I knew he was trying to preserve some dignity.

"Right here, sir," I said obediently and organized everything around his bed, within reach, next to his computer.

I left the room quickly, not wanting to embarrass him, and waited downstairs, trying to read a book. I listened for his steps to come charging down the stairs and racing into the bathroom. He didn't. An hour went by. Then another hour. And then he called.

"Mom, do you think it's done for today?"

Two whole hours! I willed that healthy team of bacteria to find nice little niches to settle into. "Sure, sweetie, go let it out."

I heard Chris calmly walk down the stairs and go into the bathroom. Two minutes later he shouted, "Having a shower."

I turned the page of my book and could feel a slow smile spreading across my face. Now we were getting somewhere.

12.

THE PROCESS

FTER THAT FIRST DAY of our new method for doing infusions, we talked about the time of day we were doing them. It was hard on Chris to do them at seven in the morning after I went to the bathroom because all he wanted to do was sleep. But that's when I went, so we had a dilemma. Because he'd been so sick for so long, it would be far better for him to sleep as much as he could. Was there any way to store the solution for a few hours?

I called Dr. Borody and asked him if one could preserve the poo for a bit.

"Well, it works best if it's fresh."

I gagged at the word "fresh." What? Were we talking about eggs?

"I think it's important that Chris sleep as much as he can, but I go first thing in the morning at about seven. He needs to sleep until about eleven."

"You can keep it in the fridge for up to six hours. But you have to cover it. Oxygen will destroy the bacteria."

"I'll put the lid on the container."

"No, no air can get to it. Completely cover it as tightly as you can with plastic kitchen wrap, like Saran Wrap or

Cling Wrap. Wrap it up. Then put on the lid, and then put it in the fridge."

Next to the lettuce, I thought. "Okay," I said.

So the next morning while Chris slept, I tightly wrapped up my you-know-what in plastic wrap, put the little package into the Tupperware and put on the lid. I tried to pretend I was wrapping up an Oh Henry! bar, saving it for later. I stuffed all this into a plastic bag and put it in the fridge. I didn't tell my friends because they'd never come to dinner.

On the second day of the new schedule, Chris slept until he naturally woke up. Then he took Gravol, a double dose of Losec, Prednisone and Imodium. He ate a little breakfast while I took my wrapped present out of the fridge and prepared the transplant. Then he squirted it in, got comfortable and played on his computer or watched movies while his feet were up in the air against the wall.

Finally, after just two days, we seemed to have it down pat.

We settled into a routine. He happily squeezed in an infusion every day, putting his feet in the air and staying like that for an hour and a half while playing on his computer. He was diligent about taking his pills all day long. He took two Imodium and two Tylenol every four hours to keep the pain and the poo at bay. He kept his rectum dosed up with steroid Anusol. He squirted in a steroid enema at night and then, after he pooed it out, took a sleeping pill. And the next morning he started it all over again. After just four nights he was sleeping for eight hours straight and I put the Ativan back in my drawer. Enough of that!

A few days later I was downstairs sweeping the floor and tidying up the kitchen when Chris yelled from the bathroom. "Mom! Mom!"

I dropped the broom and raced up the stairs. "What honey? What? Hold on. I'm coming."

I never knew what would happen next. Was he going to faint? Was he throwing up? Was he having some sort of anaphylactic reaction? I ran as fast as my legs could carry me. What if he was dying? Had cracked his skull on the bathroom sink? I burst into the bathroom, panting and dizzy with fear. Chris stood smiling beside the toilet, his hand gesturing towards the bowl, like some kind of talk show host.

I looked in, fearing the worst, my lungs burning with the exertion of dashing up the stairs. I couldn't believe what I saw.

No blood!

By the end of the first week he had stopped bleeding!

I wept, my hand on my heart. After months and months of blood everywhere it had finally stopped. He was now going to heal. My plan had worked.

We hugged each other and then reality hit us. We were admiring poo here. Chris said, "Ahem." And flushed down his first great poo in years.

Was it my plan or was it all the other medication?

Only time would tell.

The weeks went by and the snow began to melt. By the end of February, a month after the beginning of the new schedule, we started spreading the infusions out to one every second day. As Chris got better we dropped the various medications one by one. By the middle of March,

Chris was almost drug free.

The first drug to go was the green gargle. The cankers had cleared up virtually overnight so I'd stowed the bottle away under the sink in the bathroom vanity after just two days of using it. Imagine all that turmoil over a virtually instant cure for cankers.

The second thing struck off the list was the Ativan, the highly addictive anti-anxiety medication. The possibility of becoming dependent on this drug was huge, which is why I had only been given ten. I was so frightened of it I hadn't taken a single one. The last thing I wanted was my son to be addicted to tranquillizers. But after just four nights Chris was sleeping through until morning, so the bottle of six remaining pills went back into the drawer of my bedside table, waiting for another emergency. Hopefully they would never be needed again.

The Gravol had been stopped about ten days after starting it as Chris's nausea had resolved. He didn't like taking it because it made him dopey. I told him I hadn't noticed. The twenty-four hour Gravol seemed to have the worst side effect.

After about a month the deep anal fissures had healed and there were no more little foil wrappings on the bathroom floor. And we had been told only surgery would repair them. I put the remaining suppositories into a small baggie and stored them away as well.

If I'd had any extra money I would have put it in Imodium stock, I had purchased so much. But over time Chris had stopped needing it. The Imodium use had dropped from eight pills a day down to four, then down to two and then finally he was taking it as needed and then none. Chris's diarrhea was gone. I put the remainder of the package under the sink.

He hadn't been bleeding for about a month and it was time to come off the steroid enema. I read the instructions on the box and they said to taper off the doses. Hmmm, I thought, just like the Prednisone. But Chris had other ideas. Unbeknownst to me, he had simply stopped the enemas about two days before I had read the instructions.

"Mom! Mom!" Chris was shouting from upstairs.

Again I raced up the stairs. Again I didn't know what the situation was going to be. My adrenalin charged through my body like Niagara Falls. Chris was sitting on the floor of the bathroom, whiter than white and shaking like a leaf. "What's going on?" I asked him.

"I don't know. I can't stop shaking. I am so cold."

Shock?

He was curled up into a little ball, vibrating like a mal-functioning car. I ran the bath water and told him to get in and warm up. I stood anxiously outside the bathroom door, asking him every two minutes if he'd stopped shaking. Finally he said he felt better.

Back in bed, I asked him, "What was that about?"

"I think it was because I stopped taking the steroid enema."

"Oh honey, you're supposed to taper it off, like the Prednisone."

"Oops," he said.

By then it was too late to taper off responsibly, so I packed the steroid enema away as well.

Every now and then he was still popping some Losec. The two pills he was taking every morning had gone down to one and now he was taking about two a week, as needed. I kept that bottle on the kitchen counter, knowing it too would be packed away shortly. In eight weeks the tapering dose of the Prednisone would be done and that would be the last drug to go. Would we need any of these drugs again? I hoped not.

But I put them carefully into a container with a lid, just in case.

And so, by the end of March my son, Mr. Drug King, was virtually free of drugs for the first time in five years, with just the Prednisone to go. I was hopeful that this was the way it was going to be from now on, but I didn't trust it. What if his getting better had everything to do with the drugs and nothing to do with the infusions? What if the disease came back? What if he got a canker, the first sign of his infection? What would we do then?

The prospect of Chris getting sick again terrified me; were the infusions the last stop before surgery? Surely there were more options. I decided that if the infusions didn't work — which they would because Crohn's was caused by an infection, wasn't it? — I would have to accept that perhaps there was such a thing as an autoimmune disease after all.

I got back on the computer and did a little more research. I wasn't sure what to Google, but I started with "Crohn's autoimmune." I scanned down the hits and saw information on stem cell transplants! Of course! He could have a stem cell transplant. There were three places in the world where doctors were doing stem cell transplants for Crohn's disease: Spain, Italy and the U.S. This treatment was based on the theory that Crohn's was an autoimmune disease. If I had to accept that whole belief, then I would do everything I could to somehow get Chris a stem cell transplant.

We chugged along and began the third month of infusions. We were now doing them every third day! And they seemed to be working. There had been just a little random bleeding since he'd stopped after that first week of infusions. A streak here, a clot there, but nothing like the bowlfuls of blood he'd had previously. Plus, he had been completely drug free for two weeks because the Prednisone had been tapered down to zero and there was still no sign of the disease returning. I was allowing hope to settle in my heart.

Even though everything looked good, there was no way we would stop doing the transplants. That awful disease could not return. Every single MAP spore had to be killed! I pictured them hiding in unhealed edges of ulcers and deep in the folds of his intestines. I would get every last spore. The schedule wasn't that demanding and the infusions had become very easy to do. I was practiced at making up the slurry and Chris was practiced at squeezing it in. We were like a well-oiled machine. Infusions had become part of our lives.

I had a little trouble telling my friends about this wonderful treatment that we were doing for my son. I faltered every time I tried to explain the concept. We were talking about poo here! My explanation was met with everything from wise nods, to sneers, to hoots. I didn't care and neither did Chris. He was getting well. He had put on twenty pounds! He was back at the gym! He had a girlfriend! He was thinking of registering back in school! He could leave the house, walk, talk, eat! As the weather warmed up and the world was renewed, my son came back to life.

I made him sit in the spring sun, tilting his face to the warm rays. As I tucked a blanket around him I explained that tuberculosis treatment used to involve lots of sunshine, so I figured it wouldn't hurt to boost his vitamin D. I reached for his arms under the blanket and lay them on the arms of the chair, rolling up his sweatshirt sleeves so his thin arms would be touched by the sun as well. He shut his eyes and slowly moved his head from left to right, warming up his skin. As I watched him enjoying the sun I saw a rosy glow spreading over his pale cheeks. Surely this was good for him! In that quiet moment I whispered a thank you and a prayer for the future to the spirits that be. Please god, please let this work.

But even though we were now an experienced team, the infusions did have a blip or two. Every now and then one went a little awry. It wasn't always easy for Chris to hold one in. He found putting up his legs and resting his hips on a pillow helped, but as I said, sometimes there was a glitch.

Once, after an infusion, as I stood at the top of the stairs outside my son's bedroom door with a tissue in my glove-covered hand, I fondly remembered how my mother did everything she could to make me believe in the Easter Bunny. Every year the Easter Bunny brought me chocolate, some flowers, a new book. One year my mother even hand-sewed a pastel spring outfit for me and bought matching pink gloves. I was in heaven. I loved the Easter Bunny. The Easter Bunny was, in my family, placed on the same lofty plane as Santa Claus. Although my mother was an atheist, she held nothing back to manufacture for her children a living, breathing, Easter Bunny.

She left little tufts of bunny hair snagged on the edge of a table or tucked under a bed. She hid eggs in my shoes and pockets. She left pieces of nibbled carrots in corners and mangled lettuce on the stairs. She made cute little paw prints in talcum powder that she had sprinkled on the floor. She showed where the bunny had hopped by leaving trails of raisins as pretend bunny poo. Her efforts were rewarded; I completely and utterly believed in the Easter Bunny.

That day, as I stood at the top of the stairs , tissue in hand, I was reminded of all of this, but in particular I remembered the raisins. My very first thought as I went down the stairs, along the hall, and into the bathroom, was that the Easter Bunny had been eating way too much fibre. Trailing from my son's bedroom into the bathroom was a series of brown dribbles, splats if you will, that fell first onto hardwood steps, then onto carpet, then onto the bathmat and then, oh look, how quaint, to finally slide down the side of the bathtub.

Chris was in the shower.

"Hi Honey, how did your infusion go?" I asked tentatively through the shower curtain.

"Pretty good, except I had a little trouble holding it in at the end."

"Ah," I said. "You don't say."

"I'm sorry. Do you think you could clean it up?"

Now I am a good mother. A kind mother. Even a compassionate mother. Like all mothers I have cleaned up way more than my fair share of poo. What's one more drop or thirty in the ocean? "No problemo. You must have been embarrassed."

"I caught most of it," he announced proudly.

My mind boggled. "Caught" was such an interesting word. What exactly did he mean, here, in this situation?

"Oh?" I tried not to sound challenging.

"Although some landed on my rug."

I hadn't even checked his bedroom.

"What do you mean by 'caught'?"

"In the garbage pail." He said it as if I were stupid.

The shower thrummed while I tried to picture this. "What do you mean, sweetie?"

"I jetted most of it into the garbage. It was lined with a plastic bag, don't worry," he answered impatiently.

Worry? I didn't say anything. The word "jetted" flummoxed me, but then a vision of a thin, high-speed stream of shit came into my mind's focus.

"Wait," I said, "You jetted the infusion into the garbage pail? How did you do that?"

"How do you think?" His voice was sort of sneering.

I said, "Hard to say, really." I paused. "Did you aim?" I saw the stream travelling across the room at a very high velocity into his garbage.

"C'mon Mom, of course not."

"Did you sit on it?"

"That would break the pail. I held it up."

"Up? So it was closer? So you could hit it?" I couldn't get the aiming idea out of my head.

He almost shouted, "I clamped the garbage pail to my ass, okay? Get it?"

In my mind's eye I saw my son holding a very large white garbage pail to his bum, perhaps hopping on one foot, perhaps saying "yikes" and, as he put it so succinctly, jetting. I could even imagine the whoosh of sound. I knew I shouldn't laugh. It wasn't right. He was sick. He was in pain. He was dizzy. It must have been demoralizing.

I roared my head off.

When I finally got my breath I asked, "Where is the garbage pail now? On the moon?"

"Ha ha, very funny. It's in my room. The plastic bag is tied shut."

"Good thinking," I said.

13.

THE FIRST YEAR

AS TIME WENT ON and spring moved into summer, we kept doing the transplants. They were becoming less and less frequent with still no sign of the disease returning. Every three weeks I had added a day between infusions until we were doing them just once a week. We did three weeks at just once a week and then I spread out the weeks; every second week for six weeks, every third week for six weeks, until finally we were doing them once a month.

Almost a year had gone by and Chris still had no bleeding. There was not a canker, a boil, a rash, a fever, a swollen joint in sight. Did we need to keep doing the infusions? How were we to know? Maybe we could have stopped them after a month! Nobody knew. But we weren't prepared to fool around with things. All we knew was that we did not want that disease to come back.

And I knew those MAP spores were devious. They could hide anywhere.

Nonetheless, he seemed well and I decided it was time to write to Dr. Borody to tell him the good news. We hadn't connected in months and months. I wanted him to know that a most difficult case of Crohn's/colitis had been treated with fecal transplants and that the symptoms were completely gone. That we hadn't given up. I outlined in a long email how Chris had taken steroids, a steroid enema, Tylenol, Anusol, Losec, the gargle, Gravol, Imodium, and Ativan to get on a path where his intestines would stop bleeding and begin to heal so that the fecal transplant could take hold. I wrote down our lengthy infusion schedule.

I said, "The key is to not give up, to persevere. To try harder."

Two days later I heard back from him, a short capitalized message sent from his phone. He was on his way to the airport and flying to the United States. The message asked me if I would talk to some people in Boston about the treatment. A conference call at a meeting. Of course I said yes, I would do anything for the man who had told me how to save my son's life! He set up a time for the call.

I was so nervous. How could I tell a group of experts, whoever they were, about pooping into Tupperware? I mean, this was no ordinary topic of conversation.

When the time came for the conference call I was sitting at my desk, trying to stay calm. By now I knew I truly was really immature and I didn't want to guffaw so I took deep breaths as I looked out my office window. I could feel a beast of giggles uncurling in my chest, getting ready to leap up and escape, loudly. But luckily the ringing of the phone scared the laughter away and suddenly there was Dr. Borody's melodic Australian accent.

"Hi, I'm going to put you on speaker phone so everyone can hear you."

Oh great.

One by one disembodied voices asked me all sort of questions: what were the symptoms of the disease? What drugs? How many infusions? How long did it take to get a result? What was the infusion method? On and on it went. I was doing pretty well. In fact, I thought smugly, I even sounded like I knew what I was talking about. But then they wanted the nitty gritty of how this actually happened. The reality.

"How do you collect the stool?" asked an echoey voice.

I cleared my throat. I was NOT going to laugh. "In Tupperware."

I didn't say anything more and a long pause filled the long distance air.

"What size?" came the tentative question.

"The square sandwich size, only deeper. The size for storing, say, a salad."

"Oh. And why square? I would have thought round would work better."

I knew this was coming. My cheeks flamed bright red and I was grateful we weren't on Skype. What to say? I cringed and took a breath. I decided to just barrel through the truth. "No, women have to use square Tupperware so they don't get pee in the poo."

I could hear the question marks floating down the line. Finally one of the voices spoke. "Pee in the poo?"

"Yes, Dr. Borody said not to get pee in the poo."

"So," the voice paused, "How does a square shape facilitate this?"

It felt like an anvil was pressing on my chest. Was I really going to have to spell this out? Go into all the details of female anatomy? I didn't even know the right names for things.

My mind started to chant the only word I knew that had to do with female parts. A relentless "Vulva, vulva, vulva" thundered through my brain. My thoughts sounded like a backfiring engine, trying to start up. The giggling beast was starting to crawl up into my mouth from my gut. I put my head down and charged through the explanation. "Women need to tightly jam the corner of the square Tupperware in between their pee hole and their poo hole."

Pee hole? Poo hole? I sounded like I was six.

There was silence.

"I see," said the voice.

Then I heard scratching on paper. Were they taking notes? Really? Maybe they were writing down, "This lady is a nutzoid." Maybe they were writing "pee hole" and "poo hole."

Then came the next question.

"And then you scoop it into the blender, add saline, and mix up the slurry?"

Yikes. This wasn't the order. I had to explain why and how I stored it. "Actually, I have to store it for a bit until my son wakes up. I go first thing in the morning and he sleeps in. He's been sick and needs his rest."

"You store it."

"Yes."

"Where?"

Oh okay, here we go. "In the fridge."

"The fridge?" The voice sounded disgusted.

I got defensive. "I wrap it up."

"You wrap it up?"

His parroting was making me giggle. I'd held it in long enough. Laughter started to explode in my chest. I saw in my mind's eye what I thought he saw, a turd wrapped in plastic wrap lying on a shelf in my fridge. I could barely speak. A huge blasting guffaw was gathering. I tried to take deep breaths. But the image of that turd in my fridge just kept popping up. I pretended to have a coughing fit.

After it was done I said, "Excuse me. I choked on something." Yeah, my immaturity. "I wrap it up in plastic wrap so no air gets near it because that would destroy the healthy bacteria. Then I put it in Tupperware. Then I put on the lid and then I put it in a plastic bag. Then I put it in my fridge. The bacteria can't get warm because that kills them."

"So it's safe."

"Perfectly."

I was starting to laugh again. Who ever thought I'd be talking about perfectly safe poo. This certainly hadn't been one of my life's goals. I tried to regain a scientific bearing. "Then I whip it up in a blender with saline." I held the phone away from my face as I collapsed into a fit of giggles.

Dr. Borody's solid voice rescued me. "There will come a time when you'll stop doing the infusions. He is better now, isn't he?"

"Oh yes, but we can't stop. Not yet."

"Why not?"

"Well, it's like this. My son was very, very sick. Every time he sat on the toilet he pooed blood. This was very frightening. On top of all this, he was just around twenty.

This was happening when other kids his age are leaving home, going off to school, becoming young men. He completely missed a stage of growing up. To stop doing something that saved his life would be very shocking. He needs to get used to the idea that he is well. He needs to trust his body not to betray him. He will stop when he's ready to. He knows his body. He will know when the process is over. I am not going to be the person who tells him when to stop, he will tell me. He needs to feel comfortable."

I was on a soap box, I could tell, but I couldn't help myself.

"So many kids who get Crohn's either from acne medication, antibiotics, or diseased meat, are in their late teens and just beginning to be independent. They are off at school or in their first jobs and then whammo, they are struck down and totally dependent upon their parents for everything. In Chris's case, for walking even. He was utterly bedridden and had all his meals delivered. Some kids, as he was, are very close to dying. The child's normal development is grossly interrupted. The fear level is very high. I will stop doing the infusions when Chris tells me it's time to stop and not before. First of all, if the disease returns, I don't want to be blamed for stopping too early. Secondly, Chris's anxiety level has to calm down. He has to get his mind around being well."

There was silence.

Dr. Borody said, "A colonoscopy would establish how well he is. He needs one. We'll email and get one organized."

I blubbered something.

Dr. Borody continued, "Well, I guess that's all for now. Thank you Sky for talking with us."

After I hung up I filled my lungs with fresh air. An hour had gone by. I was a mess. Dr. Borody emailed me an hour later, urging me to organize a colonoscopy for Chris. He also wrote that the people he'd been talking to wanted me to be their mother. That was so nice.

But a colonoscopy? Ha ha, he'd be lucky. I knew that would never happen. Chris had already had about ten. And he'd hated every one. Getting my son anywhere near that wire snake was a pipe dream.

14.

THE COLONOSCOPY

A DAY OR TWO after the phone call with all the experts, whoever they were, Dr. Borody ramped up his crusade for Chris to have a colonoscopy. He was relentless. The emails kept coming. Finally I wrote to him saying I'd try to persuade him. This was a lie. I didn't even try. A week later Dr. Borody emailed again. He just wouldn't leave the colonoscopy idea alone.

And then he phoned. He said to me, "Tell Chris he will do a world of good."

"Okay," I squeaked. "I'll try again." Good luck with that.

But Chris had had so many colonoscopies already and he had hated the procedure. Who wouldn't? Drinking that liquid that made you poo your brains out? Going to a hospital? Getting knocked out? And then to be violated by a metal tube? Over and over again?

He flat out refused. Nothing I could say would change his mind. I even did a guilt trip. "Dr. Borody saved your life! You OWE him big."

"I'll pay him back some other way. No colonoscopy."

"Dr. Borody said you'd do a world of good."

Chris stalked out of the room. "Screw the world, it's my ass."

He had a point. It *was* his ass on the line. And given all that ass had been through, I would be protective of it as well. But I knew he had to have a colonoscopy. There had to be solid academic proof that the treatment had worked. Plus, I would feel better knowing he was well. He would feel better too. Imagine getting a great result. That would make it all concrete. He felt well and he looked well. But a colonoscopy would let us *know*.

I begged him. I pleaded. I chipped away at him until I was blue in the face. Chris said no, no, no.

Dr. Borody emailed me that a world-renowned Canadian gastroenterologist, Dr. Richard Hunt at McMaster University near Toronto, would do the colonoscopy. Together they would write an article for *The Lancet*, the famous medical journal. Chris would be the star of the article; he would be a case report!

"Tell Chris he'll be a star," he said. The pressure was mounting.

I said to Chris, "You'll be the star of numerous magazines and articles. You might just be the first one in North America to be cured of this awful disease. You'll be famous."

Chris said, "Famous? I don't want to be a famous asshole. I want to be a famous actor. Or a famous entrepreneur. Or a famous athlete. Pictures of my asshole in magazines are not part of that journey."

"Don't be stupid," I shrieked in frustration.

"No! A colonoscopy picture is not my idea of a successful man's portrait."

So, I resorted to bribery. I smiled sweetly. "What would it take for you to have a colonoscopy?"

His eyes twinkled. I could see his brain whirring. Now we were getting somewhere. I could see the little cogs in his mind fitting together. Money!

"Ah," he said, rubbing his hands together, "Forgive all my debts."

"All your debts?" I balked. He owed me for a car! Although I had bought it for him, and happily I might add because the kid couldn't walk, he had insisted on paying me back for it.

"All my debts." He was laughing. He meant it.

So I bargained. "Okay, I'll forgive the Visa bill."

I'd pay that because obviously he couldn't work and pay it off. That was a huge amount. Surely that would be enough. But he indicated with a roll of his eyes and a smirk that I had to do w-a-a-a-y more. He patted his bum and shook his head sorrowfully.

"And your cell phone bill," I added. That was another five hundred dollars. It had added up while he was downloading in bed.

He chortled derisively. Apparently he needed even more. "And the car," he chuckled.

No, not the car! Forgive the car debt? I couldn't believe it. He had been so responsible offering to pay me back for it, and here he was trying to get out of it. What a little weasel. But he just sat there, arms crossed, nodding. He jiggled his bum on the chair, just to remind me what he had to go through.

I relented. A bit. I wouldn't meet his eyes and snapped, "Okay, half the car."

He must have figured I had been pushed to the limit because he smiled and said, "Sw-e-e-e-t."

We had a deal. For thousands of dollars, the world would have a look up his bum. I emailed Dr. Borody with the good news. He was ecstatic; he'd have the evidence he needed for an upcoming conference.

A week later an envelope arrived from Dr. Hunt's office with an appointment time and instructions on how to prepare for a colonoscopy. As if we didn't know! I tossed the instructions in the garbage after making a note of the time and date. Off I went to the drug store to buy the bowel cleanser liquid. The night before the colonoscopy Chris took half of the prescribed amount saying a full dose would clean out an elephant. I didn't argue — he knew his body better than anyone.

And so it was that we were driving on the highway toward McMaster hospital in Hamilton. Chris sat stony faced beside me. "What if it shows that I am not better? What if he sees ulcers? I don't want to do this. I feel fine."

"If it shows that you have inflammation or ulcers then we'll know that you are still unwell and we will take further action." I was thinking here, "stem cell transplant."

"But I feel fine. Great. I'm strong."

"I'm sure the colonoscopy will show that you are well. You *are* well."

I could hear his teeth gritting together over the whine of the engine.

Finally the two of us were sitting in a small examination room, making jokes about poo and bums and trying to look relaxed. The doctor doing the colonoscopy came in. It wasn't Dr. Hunt, who had been struck ill. But the new fellow was great! His nametag said Dr. Ted because apparently his last name was very, very long. He asked question after question and to give him credit, never raised his eyebrows when I described whipping up poo in a blender. He assured us he would take lots of pictures and lots of biopsies. He admitted that the medical profession had just a crude understanding of intestinal diseases but that much progress had been made in the last year or two, especially in the research around genetics and autoimmune diseases.

I tried very hard not to sound impatient. In my mind's eye I saw millions of dollars flying out the window and hours and hours of good scientific minds being wasted on paths of research that would not help people. I wanted to shout to the man, "Just shove poo up people's bums! It works! They get better! Research that! Poo is the way to go!"

Instead I said, "That's interesting."

After all, the proof wasn't in yet, so how could I say anything?

The doctor went on and on about genetic predisposition, and T cells, whatever they were. I listened politely. I even nodded happily. I *was* grateful that we had this opportunity to get evidence of the success of the treatment. I *was* pleased that there would be some coordination between countries. I *was* confident that the results would be good. Chris *was* well!

So I merely said, "Well, the proof will be in the pudding." Then I turned to Chris and said, "Won't it, Pudding."

Everyone laughed and I felt the academic rhetoric fade away. Dr. Ted stood up and said, "See you in the O.R. then, in about thirty minutes."

I put my hand on Dr. Ted's arm and said, "You will be

careful, won't you? It would really be awful if, after all we've done, he got a perforation from the colonoscopy."

Now I know many doctors would be offended if their expertise was challenged, but not Dr. Ted. He was so kind and smiled at me gently. "I will do my very best. Don't worry."

My heart opened with gratitude. Here was a doctor who understood fear.

While Chris was undergoing his procedure I did what I suppose all mothers do when their children are under anesthetic. I paced. I ate. I tried to read. I ate. I walked outside. I ate. I texted friends. I prayed. I ate.

And then Chris was in recovery! I raced in and plunked beside his bed, waiting for him to wake up. Finally his eyes opened.

"Great drugs," he smiled angelically at me, his eyes loopily scanning my face.

Not the words every mother wants to hear, but hey, he was speaking! He shifted under the white sheets and let out a huge long fart. The nurse didn't even look up. He giggled with his hand over his mouth, like a two-year-old. "Sorry."

And then Dr. Ted and his resident entered the room and stood by the bed. This was it! We would know soon if Chris was better. Dr. Ted would give us a verbal report. He looked very official and serious. I searched his kind face carefully but I couldn't read if the news was good or bad. He began to talk and I sat very still, barely breathing. What would the news be?

He looked right at Chris, whose eyes were now wary slits, and said to him, "I could see from the colonoscopy that you have had a very difficult time. Your intestines are ravaged. It's been rough." The doctor's voice was soft and empathetic.

My eyes filled with tears. My poor boy. "Yes, it's been awful. He was so sick."

Dr. Ted kept looking at Chris. "I could certainly tell that from the residual scarring. I'm sorry it was so bad." He put a hand on Chris's foot and let it rest there for a minute.

I swallowed the lump in my throat and then put my chin up, I needed the verdict. I nodded at the doctor, encouraging him to continue.

"I can only give you a report based on what I could see with my naked eye. It's a visual report. The pathology results from the biopsies will come in a few weeks."

My impatience was getting the better of me. It felt as if my smile were frozen on my face. Tell me the news!!

The doctor's voice buzzed on, talking about pictures and biopsies and what have you. Yes, he said, he'd let Dr. Hunt know the results. On an on he went. Then finally he said, "My visual report concludes that there is no sign of any inflammation anywhere."

I sat up with a start. What? What did that mean? What did this doctor-speak mean? "No sign of disease?" I asked.

He repeated, "No sign of disease. No inflammation."

"Nada? No sign?" I needed to make sure.

"I saw nothing that indicates active disease."

Did I punch the air? Did I leap up and dance? Did I break down and cry with relief? I wanted to do all these things, but no, I leaned over and whispered into Chris's ear, "See? I told you so. You're a perfect asshole."

Chris smiled beautifully. "I love you Mommy." He was stoned out of his gourd. "I love you guys too," he told the doctors. He laughed.

The doctors left the area and I pulled the curtain around Chris so he could get dressed. He then wobbled towards me, grinning. "The news was good, wasn't it?"

I took his arm and guided him through the hospital hallways to the underground parking lot. No more wheelchairs for this guy. I felt as if a miracle had happened. "Yes, honey. We did it. You're better. Completely better. The news was very good."

ACKNOWLEDGEMENTS

Many people helped me on the journey to restore health to my son. I am grateful beyond words to Dr. Thomas Borody who gave his time and knowledge with unfailing generosity. Thank you also to Dr. David Baron, who saved my son's intestine and was open to fecal transplants. I will always be indebted to Dr. Mary Hanson, who was a comfort and a constant support for me throughout the often frightening experience. A heartfelt thank you to Dr. Kathleen Kerr who was kind, innovative, courageous, generous with her time, and always available. The Pharmacists at the Christie and Dupont Loblaws in Toronto always treated me with kindness, gave me the information I needed, and provided exemplary service. My friends were always there for me, laughing away and showering me with love and hope. I would like to thank John and Carolyn MacKay, who gave constant, unconditional support to me and my children throughout the years of this trying time.

In an effort to somehow repay all the help I was given, I have spent the last few years helping as many people as I could in the same way I was helped. In particular, I would like to thank these people for all they have taught me. I have learned much from them about fecal transplants and how to get them to reliably work for many intestinal diseases. These people were brave and creative, resilient and strong. As a result of my work with them, I have written *The Fecal Transplant Guidebook: Treatment for Crohn's Disease, Ulcerative Colitis, Irritable Bowel Disease. C. difficile, Constipation, Diarrhea, and More*. It is my hope that this book will help even more people who suffer from intestinal diseases become well. It is available on Amazon.com.

Finally, I would like to thank Inanna for publishing *A Gut Reaction*. I am grateful daily for Inanna's unwavering dedication to women's issues. This book is about a mother struggling, often desperately and in isolation, to prevent her child from dying by using a very unconventional method to treat his illness. Publishing a book about fecal transplants is certainly very bold and I am so grateful for Inanna's constant courage and compassion.

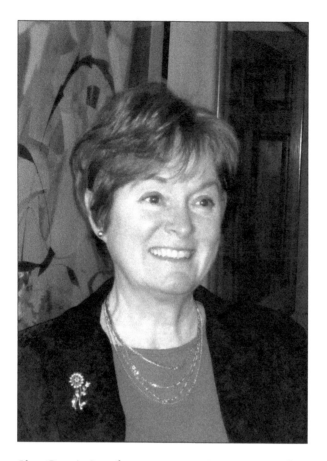

Sky Curtis is a former magazine writer, educational soft-ware designer, editor, playwright, columnist and children's writer. She now writes fiction and non-fiction books for adults. Her most recent book, *Doctored*, was published by Inanna Publications in 2010. Sky lives in Toronto with her family.